The Fine Art
of
Looking Younger

A Leading Cosmetic Surgeon's Guide to Long Lasting Beauty

by

Amiya Prasad, M.D., F.A.C.S.

Medical Director of Le Visage Cosmetic Surgery

DISCLAIMER

The information contained in this book represents the opinions of the author on a non-patient-specific basis, and should by no means be construed as the rendering of medical advice nor as a substitute for the advice of a qualified medical professional. The information contained in this book is for general reference and is intended to offer the user general information of interest. The information is not intended to replace or serve as a substitute for any medical or professional consultation or service. Certain content may represent the opinions of the author, Amiya Prasad, M.D., based on his training, experience, and observation; other physicians may have differing opinions.

All information is provided "as is" and "as available" without warranties of any kind, expressed or implied, including accuracy, timeliness, and completeness. In no instance should a user attempt to diagnose a medical condition or determine appropriate treatment based on the information contained in this book. If you are experiencing any sort of medical problem or are considering cosmetic or reconstructive surgery, you should base any and all decisions only on the advice of your personal physician who has examined you and entered into a physician-patient relationship with you.

This book is designed to provide information of a general nature about cosmetic procedures. The information is provided with the understanding that the author and publisher are not engaged in rendering any form of medical advice, professional services or recommendations. Any information contained herein should not be considered a substitute for medical advice provided person-to-person and/or in the context of a professional treatment relationship by qualified physician, dentist and/or other appropriate healthcare professional to address your individual medical needs. Your particular facts and circumstances will determine the treatment that is most appropriate to you. Consult your own physician and/or other appropriate healthcare professional on specific medical questions, including matters requiring diagnosis, treatment, therapy or medical attention. Any use of the information contained herein is solely at your own risk. Neither the author, Amiya Prasad, M.D., nor MDPress, Inc. assumes any liability or responsibility for any claims, actions, nor damages resulting from information provided in the context contained herein.

ISBN: 978–0-9792240-2-7

Printed in the United States of America.

Illustrations by Kathy Grey
Cover Design by T. Henry Litwin
Book Design by MaryRose Graphics

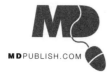

MDPUBLISH.COM   350 Fifth Avenue, Suite 7616, New York, NY 10118

ABOUT THE AUTHOR

Amiya Prasad, M.D., F.A.C.S., is the Medical Director of *Le Visage Cosmetic Surgery* with offices in Manhattan's Upper Eastside and Garden City, Long Island. Dr. Prasad has performed thousands of surgeries and specializes in Cosmetic Surgery of the eyes and face, liposuction and hair restoration. A graduate of The Mount Sinai School of Medicine in New York City, Dr. Prasad received his specialty training by top plastic surgeons associated with The University of Texas in Houston and Galveston as well as The Baylor College of Medicine. Dr Prasad is widely renowned for his innovative approach to eyelid rejuvenation and facelifting surgery. His work is highly regarded for its natural results. He has developed techniques that are well suited to modern lifestyles because he balances artistry and an individualized design with minimal risk, maximal gain and quick recovery.

He is a fellow of the prestigious American Society of Oculofacial Plastic & Reconstructive Surgery. Dr. Prasad is also a fellow of the American Academy of Cosmetic Surgery and holds board certification in Ocular Surgery as well as by the National Board of Medical Examiners.

PROFESSIONAL AFFILIATIONS

FELLOW

American Society of
Oculofacial Plastic & Reconstructive Surgery

FELLOW

American Academy of Cosmetic Surgery

DIPLOMATE

Facial Cosmetic Surgery
American Board of Cosmetic Surgery

Amiya Prasad, M.D., F.A.C.S.

61 East 66 th Street

New York , NY 10021

(212)-265-8877

Le Visage Center for Aesthetic Excellence

901 Stewart Avenue, Suite 206

Garden City , NY 11530

(516) 742-4636

www.draprasad.com

DEDICATION

To my mentors who have guided me along this amazing path to aesthetic knowledge and surgical skills, my colleagues who have pushed me to aim for ever higher ideals, my staff who enthusiastically help care for our patients, and my patients, who have made this journey worthwhile. 🐿

ACKNOWLEDGEMENTS

I would like to thank the many people who have made this book possible: my wife, Dr. Sudha Prasad, for her insightful editing, Justin James, my incredibly able Creative Media Developer for his unflagging energy in putting together the visual images, assisting with the cover design and advising on layout. I am in awe of Kathy Grey, the medical illustrator whose anatomical depictions are true works of art, and to T. Henry Litwin, the layout and cover designer for his visual design and concept for the cover. Anne Akers, our persistent publisher, who kept us on a timeline so that the book would be released on time, contributed her considerable experience and knowledge to make sure that the book progressed smoothly. My staff has been incredibly supportive and excited about the production of this book and has contributed much to the material and visual images that I was able to depict in the book.

Thanks to Dora, Joanne, Gloria, Kylene, and Sabrina for making valuable suggestions about which pictures to include. Thanks also to the Le Visage Spa staff: Barbara and Gail for their contributions to the day to day aesthetic care of our patients and for their dedication and support of our cosmetic procedures. They have proven invaluable to the patients and to me at Le Visage Center for Aesthetic Excellence for their ability to maintain and enhance the effects of the cosmetic surgery we perform.

My mentors along the way deserve special mention for their zeal to reveal to me the beauty of learning and the pleasure in pursuing self improvement. I would like to thank Dr. Penny Asbell and Dr. George Hyman for taking a chance on me way back when, Dr. Debbie Silberman, for patiently teaching me about the basic principles of surgery, Dr. Robert B. Wilkins, for showing me how to think outside of the orbit, and Dr. Russel Kreidel for instructing me in the planes of the face and the beautiful balance therein. My colleagues, Dr. Suzanne Yee, Dr. Wilbur Ha, and Dr. Robert Schwarcz have helped to provide balance and inspire me to hold my surgical skills to the highest standards.

The American Academy of Cosmetic Surgery (AACS) has been quite a forward thinking organization that is made up of some of the most interesting and talented surgeons

I have ever met, and The American Society of Oculofacial Plastic and Reconstructive Surgery (ASOPRS) have been the organizations that have provided me with professional support throughout my career.

Thanks especially to Dr. Pat McMenamin, past president of AACS, for reviewing my book in advance and providing invaluable insights.

I would like to make a special mention of Giovanni Coello, R.A. and the other talented architects at Diversified Design Associates of Huntington, NY who have created two dazzling offices that impress our patients and have remained interested and supportive of the success of the practice long after the construction ended!

I would not be able to write a book such as this without the remarkable patients that have crossed the threshold of our practice for these past 17 years and my gratitude in their confidence in me and their wise counsel is boundless.

And finally, I would like to thank my children and family for patiently tolerating my time away from them, for unflinchingly sitting by me during graphic instructional videos, and for enthusiastically contributing their opinions on the pictures and visuals for the book.

TABLE OF CONTENTS

INTRODUCTION   12

Chapter 1

Oculofacial Surgery of the Face and Eyes

A Specialist May Best Serve Your Needs   24

Chapter 2

Pitfalls of Cosmetic Surgery Today

Marketing Myths, Hype and Factory Facelifts   32

Chapter 3

Understanding the Beautiful Balance of the Face

First Impressions Say it All   62

Chapter 4

How We Age

A Decade by Decade Perspective Analysis   82

Chapter 5

The Upper Face-Superior Rejuvenation

New Innovations to Enhance Your Youth and Hasten Your Recovery   100

Chapter 6

Open Your Eyes to a New You.

An Enlightened, Less Invasive Approach
Restores Youthful Eyes   122

Chapter 7

A Better Facelift

Why the Prasad Difference Delivers   186

Frequently Asked Questions

What Patients Need to Know but
Are Afraid to Ask   212

Please Note: Color photos and illustrations
can be found on pages 129 through 160

❝The secret to a rich life is to have more beginnings than endings❞

— David Weinbaum

American Businessman and Writer

INTRODUCTION

When people ask me about my career as a cosmetic surgeon, the first thing they ask me is, "Who comes into your office? Are your clients bored, old ladies with nothing to do?" I usually reply, "I don't know anyone like that, do you?" Modern life, with its rapid forms of communication and high-speed advancement of technology, has created a swift pace of change. Some people find themselves being hauled along for the ride, and suddenly displaced. Globalization has caused many people who thought that they had a lifetime career, later arrive at the realization that they will need to find a new position. In order to accomplish that successfully, they may have to look for a way to reinvent aspects of their lives, even appearance. In fact, whether it is professional or personal, the common denominator for why people come to consult with me has very much to do with redefinition. New career opportunities, divorce, or even loss of a spouse make people sit back and reflect on their goals and ultimately rediscover their drive to move forward.

So how does one take stock of what has worked for you so far in your life? In one's twenties, people make the most of youthful attributes. They go on adventures all over the world, they invest in new business ideas, and they take pride in their appearance and attractiveness. They capitalize on sophisticated looks and style, and they live their youth with limitless possibilities. During their thirties, when adulthood hits, those carefree days become increasingly remote as responsibilities multiply and obligations abound. But as the years go by, one also may develop wisdom and the ability to make more informed choices. Life and personal relations offer deeper, richer rewards. Most of us become comfortable with who we are and what path we have chosen.

And then one day, you notice that you are perceived differently. The first time you are ever addressed as "sir" or "ma'am" is quite unsettling. You look at a snapshot of yourself and you realize that the person you see is not the same as in your mind's eye. Rationally, you admit to yourself that physical signs of aging are inevitable, but emotionally it is bewildering to accept that you would ever age.

A woman's looks, and in today's more equitable society, a man's appearance, form an important component of his or her "social capital." By social capital I refer to the ability of a person to form productive connections with others, notably friends, family, colleagues, clients, strangers, lovers, or mates. Thus our individual currency often depends on a disparate collection of variables: financial status, career, political connections, influential friends, and appearance, perhaps the most powerful and influential indicator of how we are perceived. Without saying a word, we already give strong messages about who we are — and the worth of our social capital — by our appearance. People are always judged by appearances *and age,* whether they like it or not. Once we have traveled beyond our twenties, this is a well-learned lesson for all of us.

So how does one deal with aging? Some people get on with life and never look back. I agree that a positive outlook is one of the healthier ways to live life fully. I like what Samuel Ullman suggested when he wrote his poem "Youth." He claimed, "Nobody grows old merely by living a number of years. We grow old by deserting our ideals. Years may wrinkle the skin, but to give up enthusiasm wrinkles the soul."

A passion for whatever you believe will keep you young. And I have found that those who never tire of learning, studying, and observing those around them are the ones who seem to have the most vitality. People today will eagerly stay highly active well into their senior years, perhaps remarrying or beginning a new career. Think of Martha Graham, who danced professionally until she was seventy-six, or Benjamin Franklin, who invented bifocals at the age of seventy-eight, or Georgia O'Keefe who continued painting well into her nineties. There is a good chance that in today's world you will live a long and vigorous life. Let me paraphrase what the majority of my patients tell me during our first consultation: "I'm not looking for the fountain of youth. I have it! I feel great. I just wish my appearance better matched how I feel." Others remark on working in youth culture environments, where they may erroneously be pegged as too old to dream up a creative solution. They can't change how an entire community may view aging, so their choice is quite simple. They can choose to work within that culture and perhaps turn some people's prejudice around. Or, if they choose, they can elect a simple procedure, change some signs of aging, and enhance their appearance. Either choice is correct; it must work for the individual.

Over the years, while the faces of my patients have been diverse, their needs for rejuvenation have been nearly identical. There's a common dissatisfaction with a double chin or tired-looking eyes when the patient actually feels energized, enthusiastic, and eager to engage others. Forehead lines that used to go away with a good night's rest are now deep creases. Fine lines, sun spots, skin blemishes, and sagging jowls are all subtle changes that make faces look older. My patients do not view cosmetic surgery as a panacea for feelings of low self-worth or lack of sexual attractiveness. They generally wish to look as great as they feel. That is the overriding reason people come to see me. In fact, cosmetic surgery can't possibly help the truly vain personality who derives satisfaction by seeking to feel physically superior to the rest of us. That's because there will always be another stunning woman or ruggedly handsome man just around the bend.

I have always been drawn to the beauty of the face and human body. In my spare time, I enjoy drawing, and I have spent much time analyzing the face and how its balance of features combined with the fluidity of expressions yield a truly individual face on every person. As a native New Yorker, born in New Jersey and raised on Staten Island, I always had the benefit of living in a diverse culture. I was able to study faces from all over the world. I attended City College of New York and Mt. Sinai School of Medicine, which were enriching experiences for me both personally and academically. Mt. Sinai Hospital has an international reputation, and people from all over the world sought medical care for myriad conditions, some of which were quite rare, affording me comprehensive experience.

I completed my subsequent training in eye microsurgery at Brookdale University Hospital in Brooklyn and then became an oculofacial plastic and reconstructive surgeon at the University of Texas and the Baylor College of Medicine in Galveston and Houston, Texas. I returned to my native New York planning to put my ideas about cosmetic surgery to the test. My primary interest was to bring about a natural appearance. A natural appearance means that any anti-aging change wrought upon the face in no way alters the basic character and balance that it originally possessed. Cosmetic enhancements to make the jawline appear sharper, the eyes look younger, and the neck become smoother were the types of procedures I sought to perfect.

Paramount in my goals was that I approach each individual with the sense of artistry and a respect for the balance of their face that such a tremendous task requires. Our practice began in Brooklyn and then moved on to two sites, Manhattan and Garden City, Long Island. I am quite fortunate to have found a reliable, professional, friendly, and supportive staff. Patients often remark that we seem like one big family, and in some sense we are exactly that. But there's another type of family that also heavily influences a practice: the patients. Often they will stay in touch through the years and are quite candid about how the surgery offered them a new lease on life, revealing pathways they had previously imagined to be inaccessible. As I have traveled on my journey, I have learned that cosmetic surgery can result in benefits that are both physical and emotional, both external and internal. One of the underreported consequences of successful rejuvenation surgery is that the person has a healthier appearance. People often take better care of themselves post surgery. They are more aware of what they eat, adopt new interests, or try new sports. In sum, the ramifications are immense; the new, healthy look will often lead to a fuller life.

Within the practice, we often say it is the deep and heartfelt expressions of gratitude that are most memorable. I am thrilled when patients report feeling comfortable in their clothes once again following liposuction. They participate in physical activities that they wouldn't have considered before surgery. They shop for clothes that they previously passed by because a certain kind of wardrobe would "never fit." They are no longer limited to shapeless and looser styles. Those who felt old for their years are surprised when a fresher appearance seems to open a wider circle of acquaintances. I recognize that many of these changes are actually triggered by a heightened sense of self-esteem. Yet since these benefits are quite substantial, it's difficult for me to suggest that a facelift or an eyelift can be classified as "purely cosmetic." It goes beyond the visual or superficial. In some cases, taunts from patients' youth are erased. The pain from a lost job is diminished. No longer retreating, they freely interact cheerfully with practically anyone who crosses their path.

And with renewed confidence naturally flows a new world of romance, even if it is with the spouse of decades. I'd like others who may be interested in cosmetic surgery to know that there are varied benefits to successful results. I want to offer information on how best to explore the process. The more prepared you are, the better choices you can make. A well-planned procedure can have an equally wonderful and positive influence on your life. 🐏

"Life isn't about finding yourself. Life is about creating yourself"

— George Bernard Shaw
Irish playwright

CHAPTER ONE

Oculofacial Surgery of the Face and Eyes

A Specialist May Best Serve Your Needs

culofacial. What a word, right? As one patient remarked, "How many times a day do you have to say that?" I'm not sure of the frequency, but if you haven't come across the term "oculofacial surgery" — my specialty — that's because there are only 500 or so practitioners worldwide. Specialties are exceedingly demanding, because of the extensive supplemental training required. Oculofacial surgeons must be especially mindful of the aesthetic implications of *any* tissue manipulation and the changes left behind. Like many surgeons, I tend to forget that medical terms may sound alien to patients; most medical words have roots in Latin, the language of scientists and doctors in the Middle Ages. And while that heritage continues today, most of these odd-sounding phrases are easy enough to grasp if you break them apart. For instance, *oculo* refers to the eye. The word *facial*, as a reference, is more obvious. Thus, an oculofacial surgeon is one who specializes in surgery relating to the face as well as the eye, which is an exceedingly delicate and complex structure.

In my practice, I am asked to address a wide range of challenges, and I've performed thousands of surgeries of the eyes and face. There are times when a certain oculofacial surgery will address a problem that has both aesthetic concerns and vision issues. For me, the intersection of functional and aesthetic surgery is a great source of personal and professional reward. It drives my passion. On one end of the spectrum, oculofacial surgery may improve how my patients see the world. But equally important, oculofacial surgery offers enormous potential to change how patients *are seen by the world.*

At times, this particular specialty requires me to deal in very tiny measurements, often just microns. To give you a general notion of what a micron equates to, take a look at the period punctuating this sentence. It measures nearly 400 microns. How big is the eye of an average sewing needle? Seven hundred or 800 microns wide. Dealing with fine details in this field has prepared me for the demanding requirements and varied techniques necessary to perform cosmetic surgery well. Within my specialty, I have distinguished myself as a *cosmetic* oculofacial plastic surgeon. Many of my colleagues prefer to stay in the field of reconstruction and disease management, but I have always been drawn to the cosmetic aspect of the practice, because aesthetics is a distillation of my personal lifelong interest in nature and its inherent beauty. Aesthetics demands much of a surgeon's artistic skill. The majority of my patients seek elective procedures such as eyelifts, browlifts, and facelifts.

Approximately 15 to 20 percent of my practice is made up of patients who come from all over the world for revision surgery of previous eyelifts and facelifts.

The rapid change of the rejuvenation field has extended the reach of cosmetic surgery. In fact, one could even say that today's facelift, once an exclusive indulgence for the affluent woman, now attracts a wide array of prospective patients. Some are interested in having a competitive edge in the job market. Others long for a refreshed appearance following a significant lifestyle change. For most patients, a hospital stay is no longer required. Most aesthetic procedures can be performed by qualified and fully trained cosmetic surgeons within a medical-office setting. While this is a positive trend, some people assume therefore that cosmetic surgery is like a spa treatment. But it isn't. Cosmetic surgery is still surgery.

I mention this because each day an average reader can come across a story that suggests that miraculous rejuvenation surgeries are possible during a lunchtime break. I caution readers of this book to be acutely aware that these highly publicized lunchtime lifts are built on false promises. Please do not let those late-night infomercials sway you into believing you can erase the years in an hour or so. If you read

Chapter 2, you'll understand that in reality there are no lunchtime facelifts. Heavily advertised mini facelifts today represent an unfortunate trend. No assembly line of doctors — all with varying degrees of skill and few with in-depth cosmetic training — can produce a high level of excellence, with good aesthetic results that endure the test of time.

In sum, while you may not need a specialist, I hope you will discover through a professional consultation that your surgeon is willing to individualize a solution for your needs and concerns. 🖛

"Aging is not lost youth but a new stage of opportunity and strength"

— Betty Friedan
Leader of the women's rights movement

CHAPTER TWO

Marketing Myths:

How Patients May Be Misled

If you were to name a brand, say Coca Cola, it's pretty easy to recall that product's ad or TV commercial. Advertising, especially here in the United States, is pervasive. We are surrounded by radio jingles, print campaigns and expensive, Hollywood-produced TV commercials, like those that debut on the Super Bowl. Many ads are clever, even entertaining, which is why we all seem to accept their presence. Maybe that's because a lot of ads invariably seem to imply that our current lives can be improved in some way. It doesn't matter if the ad is about a platinum charge card or a headache remedy. If we just buy that particular product or service, somehow our lives will be transformed for the better. This subtle form of persuasive selling —"try it, you'll like it"— can be convincing.

No wonder many people use advertising to shape their final buying decisions. We like to think we are all independent thinkers. But, in truth, the world of advertising helps inform our purchases, perhaps more than we care to admit. And cosmetic surgery is no exception, having been buoyed in the last decade by a significant increase in advertising. For better, and often for worse, the field has become populated with a variety of savvy, even aggressive forms of marketing.

But it wasn't always so.

There was a time when physicians and lawyers did not advertise. Any form of self-promotion was considered unprofessional, and in fact, physician advertising was against the law. Thus, if a physician enjoyed a thriving practice, much of the success was likely traceable to that doctor's reputation, which tended to flourish by referrals and word of mouth. Cosmetic surgery awareness was even more subtle, almost muted. Finding a surgeon who performed facelifts was pretty much a hush-hush discussion. Referrals were practically whispered by a trusted friend who treated the information much like a magic password. Hence, like other medical practices, a highly successful cosmetic surgeon built a practice through a network of satisfied patients who spread the word over time. A successful surgeon became, in effect, a brand.

Advertising: Beauty and the Beast

While American physicians were forbidden to advertise, plastic surgeons in South America and Mexico flourished via splashy advertising and expensive public relation arrangements. Their marketing efforts were so successful that our national media began to cover their marketing techniques. TV stories focused on the "bargains" one could enjoy south of the border.

Soon, Americans were jumping on planes and flying to Rio for all sorts of nips and tucks. The results, however, were mixed.

The switch to marketing a medical practice via advertising materialized in the 1980s, a decade when certain industries were deregulated. Reins were loosened on banking institutions, and it became legal for physicians and lawyers alike to advertise. With physicians finally being able to *legally* advertise here in the States, the world of cosmetic surgery was completely recast. At times the transformation has been for the better. The general public could read more about emerging technologies as the veil of secrecy was removed. The beauty of the early days of advertising is that it stirred a genuine interest in the field.

No longer the exclusive choice of the society matron or movie star, advertising democratized cosmetic surgery. But the beastly aspect to advertising is that frequently claims and promises have been overstated. Before and After photos have been and continue to be "doctored." Quickie procedures, often touted as effective and long-lasting as other more traditional aesthetic surgeries, attracted the naïve; many were left disenchanted. Through increased consumer demand, doctors in fields other than cosmetic surgery, with declining practices, recognized a gold mine. Many could simply take a weekend seminar, hang out a sign, slap a fancy-looking certificate on the wall, and be in "the cosmetic surgery business" within days. There was the added incentive of no insurance forms, since cosmetic surgery is elective.

Still, many reputable physicians did advertise legitimately and built thriving practices by credible use of marketing.

My Foray

Not wanting to mislead prospective patients, I thought I had stumbled upon a meaningful way to communicate my point of difference. A few years ago, several of my patients remarked on their quick recoveries and other benefits. Within their circle, they knew friends or family members who had used other surgeons — all top names and excellent physicians — but the results from the other surgeries seemed to entail longer periods of downtime. There also appeared to be more post-operative bruising. With other surgeons, even the incision marks seemed to be longer. For the most part, general anesthesia was used by these other top surgeons, *not the local anesthesia I prefer*. "Your facelift is smarter," offered one patient, and as soon as she blurted the words out, I had a small epiphany: Why not call my approach The Smart Lift? Every day I witnessed how quickly patients bounced back. The process was smarter. They returned to normal routines after less downtime and enjoyed beautiful long-lasting results. Done. I decided to use the name: SmartLift.

However, it wasn't too long before I came to appreciate why no single brand name could possibly sum up an individualized approach to each patient. As I welcomed new patients, we would consult about their expectations. I discovered that some patients were confused. They wanted to know how my SmartLift differed from other branded facelifts. I wondered: What "other" branded facelifts? Some would ask: Was my approach like the ones they saw on a late-night TV infomercial? How about that print ad with an 800 telephone number? I remember pausing to ask myself, "What have I done?" How could my years of expertise ever be packaged as a mass-marketed branded facelift? If American patients were confused, what would my international patients think? So there it was: Even I was seduced by the implicit power of advertising.

At that time, my practice had made a quantum leap, and the days for my employees and me were exceedingly busy. Still, I forced myself to pause and "mentally regroup." With my private practice, I have always sought to raise standards. I spend a good deal of time with consultations — perhaps more time than most top surgeons. That's part of my reputation: Thorough, one-on-one time with new patients, who must never feel rushed. Longer consultations benefit me as well. I really have to understand what each patient hopes to achieve in order to deliver the results he or she seeks. Plus, I enjoy interacting with individuals, simply because each person is unique.

Over the years, as I built a successful practice, I viewed our post-operative care to be among the best in the world. I pride myself on hiring the most wonderful, compassionate and capable support staff. We are a team, and together we all keep the practice and offices humming like a rare Stradivarius. It may sound corny, but to most patients we are a happy family. We really are. And that's when I had the second, even more important epiphany: If we were family, how could we be a mass-marketed brand? The answer is that we can't be. I saw no reason to continue with my SmartLift brand name. This well-intentioned foray into marketing was left to quietly expire on its own.

Nevertheless, I do remain curious about how others market cosmetic surgery. Since the field continues to attract a wide cross-section of physicians, many with varying levels of skill, exactly how do today's doctors develop a practice? The answers are as diverse as the doctors themselves.

As a surgeon, I understand that the medical world can be intimidating for some people; many patients simply abdicate to the doctor. I was the eldest child in my family and felt a personal obligation to act on my parents' behalf when chronic illness flared up. Any child would naturally assume, "These doctors have gone to medical school. They know what they are doing." Actually, in my case and at that time, there was a certain truth and logic to this thinking. But today, and in your case, when it comes to exploring cosmetic surgery: Be your own advocate. Be adult about your surgery. Stay involved. Don't acquiesce. Do your homework. Average consumers do more research when buying a car or a computer than when choosing a physician. That's typically because most people do not know how to compare physicians, how to research their background and what questions to ask. But in this chapter, you'll learn how to avoid the pitfalls of cosmetic surgery. I've written an addendum to the book on how to decipher fancy-sounding credentials and how to screen surgeons to find the best candidate. Let me share what I have observed and what I have learned.

Caveat Emptor

The Latin phrase caveat emptor translates to "Let the buyer beware." The idea is that buyers take responsibility for what they are purchasing. It's important to do a little research. If the promise appears too good to be true, well, then, perhaps it is. Physicians are human. All doctors vary in quality and expertise due to a number of factors, but four differences are key: ability, training, experience, and service.

In the *Introduction* I touched on my training at Mt. Sinai Hospital. I know it made me a better physician, because patients arrive there from the world over in large numbers, and the challenges are varied and omnipresent. I would never see the wide swath of unique conditions, complex issues, and sheer numbers if I were in a small city or rural area. In a week, my hospital receives more patients and interesting cases than many facilities might see in an entire year, though to be sure, there are many wonderful and highly qualified facilities and top physicians across the country, in cities large and small.

Credentials and Experience

Analyzing a doctor's credentials may be confusing. Here's how to keep it simple. If you opened a car door and slid into the passenger seat, you'd like to know that the person behind the wheel had a driver's license, right? In order to get that license, the person passed a standardized test — was able to read the road signs and observe the laws of the road. That's what a driver's license signifies. And for those who break the rules and get caught, licenses are flagged. Repeated offenders lose their license. It's pretty much the same for doctors when reviewed by licensing boards

Remember the phrase "caveat emptor"? You *must* protect yourself, and it's important to understand that a doctor's credentials go beyond state licensing and can be quite varied.

Here are the areas worth researching:

Education. What school did the doctor attend? What year did he or she graduate? Education will include medical school, residency, and fellowship training, if any and it's a good place to begin.

State Medical Licensing. Licensing varies by state, and you can access a quick, state-specific medical licensing board via the Internet. This should produce the appropriate licensing group to contact. Most state licensing boards are accessible by telephone, which should be listed on each state's website.

Additional Certifications. Because medicine is so complex, additional certification may include board certification or qualifying exams for doctors to become members of elite, superspecialist groups. If you need to understand further how to sort through the credentials your doctor tells you about, seek clarification by asking the doctor directly what each certificate means. Make sure you find out what type of specialized training the surgeon has completed. If the answer is none, it's wise to interview another surgeon with a specialization so you can better determine whose skill best fits your aesthetic goals.

Experience. Obviously this varies by each individual surgeon and remains a difficult area to quantify and appreciate. Clearly, strong word of mouth from a variety of gratified patients whose results appear natural and aesthetically pleasing offers some basis for choice. You may also learn how to effectively read Before and After pictures, winnowing out those that disguise inconsistencies with lighting and makeup.

The background, lighting, level of makeup, and other variables should be consistent and equal across both images. It may also be worthwhile to quantify how often the doctor performs the type of procedure you are interested in.

Non-Hospital Surgery. Some states require medical offices that do surgery on site to be accredited. This safety review establishes standards to protect the patient in much the way hospitals must meet standards. Official on-site inspections for safety, efficiency, and appropriately qualified personnel are made by an outside organization. Many stringent standards must be followed in order to maintain accreditation. Many practices are required to provide accreditation letters to patients who ask for proof; practices who have passed inspection post certificates so that patients may easily read them when visiting an office. If you want to know if your state requires accreditation, do an Internet search before your consultation.

Specialty-Based Organization Memberships.

A plethora of professional organizations (and unfortunately, organizations that sound professional but may not be) often make it challenging for a new patient to learn about the surgeon and the practice. For patients seeking a specialist in facial rejuvenation, I recommend two sources.

AACS. The American Academy of Cosmetic Surgery is an Illinois based, not-for-profit professional medical society whose members are dedicated to patient safety and physician education in cosmetic surgery. Most members of AACS are facial plastic surgeons, head and neck surgeons, oral and maxillofacial surgeons, dermatological surgeons, varied plastic surgeons, and ocular plastic surgeons — all of whom specialize in cosmetic surgery. AACS is the organization that represents cosmetic surgeons in the American Medical Association through its seat in the AMA House of Delegates.

— *www.cosmeticsurgery.org*

ASOPRS. Founded in 1969, the American Society of Ophthalmic Plastic and Reconstructive Surgery is a body of qualified surgeons who have training and experience in this highly specialized field. The purpose of ASOPRS is to advance education, research, and the quality of clinical practice in the fields of aesthetic, plastic, and reconstructive surgery specializing in the face, orbits, eyelids, and lacrimal (tear duct) system.

The Society, located in Minneapolis, has more than 550 national and international members. It sponsors several annual high-level scientific conferences and seventeen national fellowships for top postgraduate physicians who have completed an accredited ophthalmology residency. This is a very select group of surgeons who withstand a great deal of competition in order to get one of these fellowships. The site offers a section listing surgeons by geographic location.

— *www.asoprs.org*

In sum, do your homework. Some patients tend to dismiss the possibility of cosmetic surgery complications. They assume that the surgery is merely aesthetic, thinking, "It's elective and not life-threatening, right?" Again: Caveat emptor. Cosmetic surgery is still surgery; your body does not know the difference. You owe it to yourself to choose the surgeon who will deliver your aesthetic results safely.

One Size Fits All: Pitfalls of Pit-Stop Face Lifts

Today, mass-marketed facelifts continue to proliferate as companies, not necessarily individual surgeons, seek to capitalize on consumer interest. One of my patients invented the perfect phrase to describe this trend: "factory facelifts." Unfortunately, due to late-night infomercials and extensive print campaigns, the general public is beginning to equate these surgeries with quickie spa treatments. The result is the public is continually being misled. First, the Before and After photos of these infomercials suggest that a "one size fits all" lift can uniformly reverse signs of aging. In truth, no one single approach can possibly work uniformly across a general population. Each face is a complex system of skin, tissue, and muscle that comes together in a highly unique expression of a single person.

A face reflects a person's distinct character. There really can't be a "one size fits all" facelift. If I were rejuvenating your twin sister or brother, the steps I would take would be remarkably different than steps to rejuvenate your face, since the underlying structure is only one of the many considerations I must examine. I must also consider a patient's lifestyle, the toll of stress over the years, extent of sun exposure, smoking habits, if any, and underlying medical status. No two people are alike. In a factory facelift system, however, these nuances can't possibly be addressed with great skill and finesse in order to consistently deliver satisfactory results.

Your best bet is to avoid a company that seeks to mass market cosmetic surgery, using a behind-the-scenes coterie of physicians. A cosmetic surgery company offering brand-name facelifts really is no different than an automotive assembly line. It cannot deliver the type of long-term, aesthetically pleasing results that are best offered by a single, specifically trained specialist, an expert at determining each person's needs.

Unfortunately, what most prospective patients take away from these infomercials is a soft sell of a quasi beauty treatment, much the way cosmetic companies over the year have sold "hope in a jar" with beauty creams. Again, if it looks too good to be true, it probably is. Remember the value of a specific surgeon's credentials: Any number of physicians who participate in a mass-marketed facelift program may become "overnight experts" by taking a one- or two-day seminar. In fact, your surgeon could be a family practitioner who is seeking to add a stream of income.

In sum, a large production facility may be effective for manufacturing computers or any product that must conform to uniform specifications to meet buyer standards. It's an ineffective system, however, for conducting aesthetic surgery. And in many cases, this assembly line system has all the potential for creating lopsided, unacceptable, or even dangerous results.

Exactly what is a mass marketed facelift anyway? I recall waiting in an airport, thumbing through an issue of *Family Circle*, when I came across a print ad for what I thought was a simple beauty treatment with spa overtones. But as I read the copy, I learned that the product was actually a surgical facelift. The copywriter gave the procedure a branded name and the approach resembled a day spa treatment that was both innovative and "revolutionary." In fact, this very procedure has been discussed at any number of high-level medical conferences, where the experts concluded that the approach is identical to what now is popularly known as a mini lift. The mini lift is a type of surgical procedure that earned some press in the early 2000s but has fallen out of favor today. Why? *The mini lift produces mini results.* For all its introductory fanfare, for all its highly touted benefits and inflated revolutionary outcomes, the mini lift failed because it could not deliver meaningful results. The rejuvenation was short-lived. That's why most reputable surgeons can't possibly build a successful practice by offering only mini lifts.

The ad copy suggests that "wrinkles, frown lines and sagging skin" are removed in about an hour. An hour? You and I can't get through airport security in an hour. What that hour *really* implies is quick patient turnover, much like the need to flip tables in a restaurant enjoying an overnight surge in popularity. How satisfying can that type of dining experience be? Is the quickie surgery about delivering a high level of personal care? Is it about careful post-operative supervision? Or is it more about flipping tables or patients?

Obviously, the more patient traffic processed in a shorter time frame, the more profit for the company. So perhaps you're reading the ad and think, "Wow. An hour and I'm done!" But view the promise from the company's angle: They need to make a profit; they need quick turnover. You — and the rest of the patients on the assembly line — had best be moving in and out at a fast pace, no matter what your unique situation presents. To me, any cookie cutter or one-size-fits-all approach inherently trivializes surgery. It almost equates surgery to a manicure or a beauty makeover by a fashion stylist. No surgery, including aesthetic surgery, can be reduced to a "spa-like" pit stop. Further, all faces are unique. Each face has its own balance of features and skin type as well as skin tone. No mass-marketed facelift can effectively work across a wide population using one approach and yet uniformly deliver meaningful, individualized results. How can an hour — or as the ad puts it, "about" an hour — possibly deliver an effective rejuvenation outcome, one with beautiful and long-lasting results? It can't. Again, if the claims in the ad sound too good to be true, they probably are.

Other nationally marketed cosmetic packages also promote stellar results using local anesthesia, requiring a short recovery. In this case, a parent company is the marketing force that pays for the expensive television commercials and print ads and then spreads the sales leads across its base of partner physicians, taking a fee for the referrals. In some cases, these physicians do have their own practices and may offer their own traditional facelifts too. But they participate in these ad campaigns and pay referral fees because their practice needs a boost. If you think about this new type of marketing as a hard-core business venture, the high cost of advertising also dictates that a high percentage of leads must be quickly converted into sales. No surprise then, that the pressure is applied to prospects as soon as they make a preliminary inquiry. What I found disturbing is the role that consultants play within these business ventures. Prospective patients meet with *consultants*, not surgeons. If you were to come to my office for a visit, what good would a consultant do? So I had to wonder: How does one become a cosmetic surgery consultant anyway? No surprise: Consultants are recruited through any number of Internet employment ads, like those on monster.com. Consultants are salespeople. Their job is to convert *you* into a *sale*.

A *New York Times* article reported that facelift franchise consultants may employ high-pressure sales tactics to get you to sign up. But the medical field recognizes that any form of a hard sell is inappropriate to cosmetic surgery. If you're ever in a physician's office or exploring a facelift franchise and feel you are being pushed to get a facelift, get up and leave. No reputable surgeon employs this kind of tactic. In the same *New York Times* article it was evident that prospects often don't meet with surgeons as part of the general routine, *even before surgery!* And the real spin of these assembly line companies is price: Most tend to fall in the $4,000 to $6,000 range, which is an impractical bargain-basement price for a facelift. As a disappointed patient summed up her assembly line experience to me: "My results were so disappointing, I received virtually nothing for my money." I often ask my patients this: "Do you really want a bargain for your *face?*"

Individual Physician Ads

Advertising has provided a means for some physicians to build instant reputations. However, since advertising is expensive, there has to be some selectivity, some process to winnow out those prospects who may not need surgery or may have unreasonable expectations. Assembly lines, however, are designed to keep the product moving through the system, so few patients are ever disqualified. Yet, as a cosmetic oculofacial plastic surgeon, on occasion I have detected underlying medical issues pertaining to patients seeking a simple eyelift. Without proper screening, there may be a series of unsatisfactory results or an increase in post-operative problems. More important, there may be a missed diagnosis of an underlying disease. For instance, *ptosis*, or drooping of the upper lid, is often the precursor of myasthenia gravis. In these instances, a neurologist must be consulted. One can't presume an assembly line will make the distinction between natural aging and ptosis triggered by a more serious condition.

Advertising has the potential to imply quality where there is none, or to embellish credentials. Again, confirm the surgeon's credentials. Research the physician's reputation. Do not rely on an ad that exaggerates success or expertise. Find former patients and speak with them; probe them about their consultation and level of attentive post-operative care. And really scrutinize Before and After photos for accuracy. See if you can determine if the lighting has changed or if makeup skews reality.

Also, all surgery has risks. Ads that offer unrealistic expectations, devoid of qualifiers, are suspect. For example, if an ad says "Look ten years younger right away!" or "The only facelift that will take years off your face instantly," these are highly exaggerated claims that make no allowance for special circumstances. They couldn't possibly be true. Finally, beware of ads that speak of "new" or "revolutionary" techniques. For the most part, if something is truly new or revolutionary, *let others test it.* With skilled physicians, there are no overnight magical tricks. The majority of excellent results come from time-tested methods, many of which have been updated and refined — perhaps streamlined and improved — by innovative surgeons. From these innovators, new techniques help refine aesthetic results, often traceable to the special ability of the surgeon alone. New methods evolve and advance with time. There are no overnight miracle cosmetic surgery breakthroughs, despite what many infomercials and expensive marketing campaigns suggest.

As ad spending increases, be aware that more cosmetic gimmicks in the future will seek to break through the clutter. The net of cosmetic surgery marketing is thrown to a wider audience. Over time, a greater proportion of the public increasingly falls under its spell. Be wary of cosmetic surgery featured in lengthy infomercials, similar to those for a kitchen gadget or a miracle laundry powder, or an exercise swivel chair that reputedly can cinch your waist muscles in minutes. This premise is worth restating: Cosmetic surgery is still surgery. It is not a gadget or a widget. No physician can take a wand and magically wave away years with an easy, fast, lunchtime pit stop.

Celebrity Physicians, Social Doctors, and Publicity

Pick up a newspaper and there it is: a headline story on cosmetic surgery. Turn on your television just about any time and you'll find a news show or lifestyle program about cosmetic procedures. TV shows, both reality and fictional, as well as popular magazines such as *People*, provide the latest gossip on who's been nipped. And tucked. Even the more affluent publications, such as *Town & Country* and Vogue, do round-up articles on leading doctors and what's new in the cosmetic world.

I personally have benefited from a few of these stories. Again, I like speaking with people, and I am often available to speak with the press. I've been on local TV and in national journals and consumer magazines alike. However, sometimes it seems that some reporters read stories and develop a base of "experts" by simply drawing on the same contacts year after year. This leads to me to two small publicity "catches" I'd like you to be aware of.

Media Buzz

First, magazines, TV — all forms of media, including the Internet — have an ongoing need for content in order to survive. They have to fill their pages or air time with information. For that reason, some of the coverage may not indicate a true trend, actually qualify as "news," or be noteworthy. "Story inventory" has to be filled. Should you come across a TV segment that supposedly is covering a cosmetic surgery breakthrough, quite possibly the "innovation" came from a doctor's publicity agent, who simply pitched the idea to a producer.

Celebrity Following

Second, in big cities, such as New York, Los Angeles, and Chicago, good physicians can quickly develop a following of important, influential people whose names are often bold-faced in society columns. You read about their comings and goings in the social scene in Paris, the Hamptons, and so forth. In full disclosure, I admit that I have my share of influential patients, though I work very hard to treat all patients equally. Tycoons, movie stars, and heiresses do not necessarily earn longer consultations, though often they must be seen and treated outside of normal office hours. Still, I work very hard to develop a practice that has a wide cross-section of patients, including those from abroad. I do not want a practice built on celebrities and bold-faced social names. I need to take time to think about my techniques, and the hype that comes with dealing with high-profile figures is an extra layer of distraction that keeps me from taking those creative breaks that permit me to reflect. Surgeons must be able to put aside time to explore innovations and grow personally.

Much like in my early days as a young intern, I am always searching for a better way. If I have the chance to raise the level of an accepted standard, I will strive to make it a reality. Yet if I am constantly seeking the buzz of publicity, then I can become quickly overbooked and transform my practice into a veritable treadmill. When would I have time to meet with peers, colleagues, and true medical innovators as a means of personal growth? So I see a liability for average patients who seek out the "big name" surgeons expecting amazing results. Treadmills don't produce amazing results. Some of the prominent Beverly Hills and Park Avenue surgeons deprived themselves of a real chance to grow. Instead, they sought the publicity wave and found the ride entertaining for a while, only to later realize they were bound by the more conventional and traditional surgeries as a means to stay afloat. A practice built on celebrated patients diminishes a surgeon's time and energy to improve, to innovate.

Don't rely only on the name of a surgeon mentioned in a popular magazine to persuade you. Look beyond the TV appearance. Don't rely only on *a* print article, such as those with the headline "The Top Cosmetic Surgeons." I don't wish to suggest that a doctor's publicity is wrong. Having a bit of publicity can generate greater awareness, and as awareness grows, the general public benefits. In fact, I have benefited from this press, and it is a nice addition to any practice. In the end, however, publicity is transitory, and somewhat like glory, fleeting. Experience is long-lasting and leaves a legacy, and it is worth the effort to seek it out. 🐦

"Everything has beauty, but not everyone sees it "

— Confucius

Chinese thinker and social philosopher

CHAPTER THREE

Understanding the Beautiful Balance of the Face:

First Impressions Say It All

When it comes to expressing how we feel, words alone can communicate just so much. Real pain and joy are more vividly expressed by the face. That's why the human face is called our most important "communication tool." Our face is a dynamic canvas, one on which emotions appear in undeniable clarity and then instantly evaporate. As we mature, reading faces becomes second nature. Yet failing to read emotions correctly — or sending the wrong facial cue ourselves — may compromise our effectiveness with family, friends, colleagues, and strangers. Understanding faces is part of our human DNA: newborn infants show a noticeable predilection for the human face above all other objects. If you doubt the importance of the face, think about a child's drawing of a family member. Invariably, the face is disproportionately bigger than the rest of the body, resting like a globe on two spindly legs. In sum, our face is pivotal to who we are, a social ID tag of sorts.

I hope you'll pause in the coming days to study faces: yours and others. The reason for this exercise is simple. Most adults are reasonably sophisticated at reading other people's expressions. But in this chapter, I'd like you to consider "micro expressions." These are the imperceptible expressions that contribute to our character and sense of identity. Why is this important? When we think of rejuvenation, the tendency is to focus on the signs of aging and how to best eliminate them. However, in the process, you don't want to diminish special appealing, expressive nuances that make you unique. Without those wonderful individual expressions that distinguish you from the rest of the world, a desirable part of your identity may be irretrievably lost.

If you are considering any type of anti-aging procedure — from fillers to Botox to a facelift — I urge you to seek the surgeon who is best able to *preserve your own beautiful identity* while diminishing those aging signs you find troublesome. If you don't, you may find yourself lamenting, "I don't look like myself anymore." This is a serious and increasing problem of inferior cosmetic surgery: unskilled procedures inadvertently compromise character by removing important elements of an individual's special beauty.

How does the problem of "overcorrection" arise? One of the ironies of life is that certain expressions, those that make a person unique, may also cause the face to age. Yes, happy people laugh a lot. And some get laugh lines. Patients who are blessed with sparkling eyes and a zest for life may be frustrated when these cheerful expressions give way to a look of fatigue —

even though they've never felt better! Frequently, patients speak of being at the "top of their game." At a time when peak performers should be reaping all the rewards of hard work, certain aging signs seem to detract from the face they present to the world. Excited about their careers and life, they often realize that the mirror's image doesn't reflect the vitality they *feel*. They look weary.

I'd like to share two cases with you. First, one beautiful client, immediately following a new business pitch, was questioned about her ability to take on a new and progressive client. Her creative pitch was far superior to those of her competitors. But the client team, through informal discussions with others, made the staff aware that perhaps she may have been "too old" for their innovative account. Might she be ill equipped to supervise younger teams? When she first heard this reaction, I think she was truly crestfallen. But by the time she came to me, she said, "I really can't change how the world thinks, can I? Maybe I should just tweak my appearance a bit." Neither of us felt a radical correction was needed. Instead, she would benefit from a facelift in order to appear more refreshed and energized. In the end, her outward appearance simply reflected exactly how great she felt inside: excited about life and able to contribute significantly to new business growth!

Another client, a lighthearted man, was often asked, "What's wrong?" For a long time he just didn't understand the question. Over time, as the frequency of the same question increased, he had to wonder, "What mixed signals am I sending?" Thriving in his job, he was the best at handling high-volume client demands that resulted from critically important scheduling issues. Where seemingly impossible deadlines were the status quo, he was skilled at providing innovative solutions. Yet his ongoing problem solving — and deep thoughts — showed up on his forehead, an expressive focal point for many people. We know the phrase "beetle-browed" connotes a bad-tempered or surly person. Yet this patient was a great guy, good-tempered and pleasant. You just couldn't tell that by his appearance. His forehead was a tangle of lines and furrows. That's why customer feedback pegged him wrong: He was often referred to as looking depressed, even angry. Although one cosmetic surgeon suggested a browlift, in his case, this seemed extreme. Yes, a browlift might eliminate those unsightly furrows. But a brow lift would likely change his appearance beyond what was necessary. Instead, simple Botox injections were all that was needed to maintain the integrity of his personality and erase his worried look.

These are two simple examples to illustrate that your face is an important agent of identity, a mirror of your emotions and a barometer of your attitude. You may wish to diminish signs of aging, but it's critically important to protect the integrity of those desirable and beautiful expressions that make you unique. Our face develops as we do, from infancy into the teen years and adulthood, through our middle-aged years, and finally into the senior years — always retaining those individual features originally prominent in childhood. We all age, but our faces define who we are. The challenge for any skilled surgeon *is to rejuvenate, not create a new person.*

Apart from identity, the face provides vital clues to an impressive variety of possibilities: attraction, age, sense of humor, and personality. In addition, faces reveal a person's mix of ethnic origins. In fact, the face is perhaps the most important art object throughout time and from all civilizations. Most of us can re-imagine the face of the boy Egyptian king Tutankhamen or the smile of the Mona Lisa or Vincent van Gogh's red beard. We have learned fascinating properties of genetics that help shape the modern face. Many anthropologists are quick to point out that there is no such thing as a specific face that belongs to one particular race. We have all become blended in our appearance as new and intriguing combinations arise with each generation. A face can signal success, even social rank, and how well the person is able to connect with peers and superiors. The face also functions as a "mating" billboard of sorts. When it comes to selecting a partner, there is a broad societal assumption, that more attractive, symmetrical body types and faces tend to make higher quality mates. The rationale behind symmetry preference in both humans and animals, is that symmetric individuals are thought to be healthier, less riddled with disease and have fewer genetic defects. Thus, a symmetrical face, on an almost subliminal level, is suggestive of more robust genes, improving the likelihood that an individual's offspring will survive. Understanding sex-specific facial differences also illustrates another intriguing way that the human face serves as a tool when searching for a mate.

Male and Female Facial Attributes

From our earliest days, differences between male and female faces emerge. A baby's boy head tends to be bigger, and as both sexes move toward maturity, the female skull tends to grow to about two-thirds the size of the male on average. The female head also has smaller ridges of bone on the jaw and brow. Males are likely to have larger, longer and wider noses. In part this is traceable to males generally being bigger — a larger nose permits more air to be inhaled into larger lungs in order to carry around a larger frame. And other sex-specific differences prevail. That makes sense: if there were no differences, how else might we differentiate prospects for procreation? At puberty, a male's skin toughens and becomes coarser due to hormones that make pores expand and facial hair sprout. While male eyebrows are thicker, women have more fat on their cheeks, giving a softer facial outline. In fact, the appearance of high cheekbones really is generally more about the way facial fat is distributed and less about actual bone structure.

Toward adolescence, a young woman's lips appear fuller than those of male peers. Since women's faces do not have as much bone mass as men's, female eyes often generally appear more prominent. Structural variables explain why. First, while the eyeball is nearly the same size in both men and women, women's eyes appear larger because female eyebrows are generally higher up. And since a woman's forehead typically appears more upright and slight, this facial combination makes females' eyes appear larger. Women's facial muscles are smaller, and female facial fat hides muscles better.

All human facial expressions are built upon this foundation of bone and flesh. The appearance of the face is formed by the shapes and placement of the bones of the skull, the cartilage, and the soft tissues, including the muscles, fat, and skin and the facial features they form. Despite the advancement of years, a human face, say that of an eighty-year old woman, will nearly always retain features already prominent in childhood. *But expressions make us who we are.*

Expressions

The emotional human face permits us to recognize common expressions such as happiness, curiosity, surprise, or anger in others. In people we know a bit better, we can spot subtle emotional nuances such as disappointment, fatigue, or boredom. There appears to be a genetic component to human facial expressions; we are most likely born with the ability to express emotions — they are hardwired to our brains, rather than learned. How do we know this? A number of studies have explored the statistical correlation between facial expressions of sighted and blind individuals. Guess what? Without seeing the faces of others, the expressions of blind people mirror those considered identical to universal emotions and feelings.

Still, science seems to go back and forth, testing to see if the five basic emotions — happiness, surprise, anger, sadness, fear, disgust/contempt — are the same the world over. The research is complex, but for the purposes of this book we can agree that expressions around the globe are about the same. However, newer research also underscores that cultural differences do exist. There are parts of Asia, for example, where strong emotional displays are discouraged. Also, eyes may be lowered during a simple conversation; it's a way to show respect, since continued direct eye contact could signal an overzealous sense of competition. Thailand is often called the "Land of Smiles," and with good reason. In that country, a smile is the most appropriate reaction to difficult situations. Lose a wallet? Hotel has no record of your reservation? Thais will likely smile at your anxiety, which tends to frustrate Americans who assume that a smile means indifference. But in general, human facial expressions, and how we collectively react to situations, clearly indicate that a universal language of emotions prevails. If you've ever watched the news and seen the faces of survivors following a tsunami, you recognize that grief, despair, and anxiety look much the same in remote regions as anywhere else.

You Be The Judge

As the old saying goes, you can't judge a book by its cover. But people do it all the time! So, how much do you know about the human face? Are the eyes the most significant aspect to a person's beauty? Before we briefly touch on facial aging — other chapters explore the subject more extensively — why not take a quick quiz to show much you know about certain facial basics? Perhaps some of the answers may surprise you.

1. The human nose defines the human face.

    a. True

    b. False

2. The key facial features of the two sexes are nearly the same, distinguished only by size — men's features generally are larger.

    a. True

    b. False

3. Which feature generally plays a larger role in a person's attractiveness?

    a. Lips

    b. Nose

    c. Eyes

d. Cheeks

e. Chin

f. Face shape: oval, square, or round

4. Which facial area first shows signs of aging?

a. Eyes

b. Mouth

c. Lips

d. Cheeks

5. Which description fits the ideal shape for a woman's eyebrow?

a. Full and flat with a gentle curved shape

b. Thin, somewhat flat with a gentle curved shape

c. Full and straight, a classic line

d. A high arched shape that tapers

6. Gravity is a significant contributor to aging. You can't fight it. Over time, it just pulls facial structure downward.

a. True

b. False

7. The most important factor that determines how well a person ages is:

    a. Little or no sun damage

    b. Amount of volume in the mid face

    c. The absence of crow's-feet

    d. No sign of bags and/or dark circles under the eye

How well did you do?

1. False – The face is a collection of features that gives a person his or her own identity; even if a nose is proportionately larger than other features, the nose does not define the human face.

2. False – While men's features tend to be larger, a variety of sex-specific variables make the male face different from a woman's. Generally, softer curves and facial plumpness distinguish the female face, while the male face is more angular. Men are often considered "ruggedly handsome," with cheeks that are short, narrow and prominently placed on the face.

3. D – The cheeks generally determine if a face will appear masculine or feminine, youthful or old — and thus they account for much of a person's perceived beauty. To be sure, youthful or plump cheeks can help frame beautiful eyes, which may appear to be the focal point. But in the absence of a soft cheek area, even beautiful eyes can appear wan or weary.

4. A – The eyes begin to show signs of aging as we approach our third decade. Certain tissues begin to sag, and the outer portions of the upper eyelids lose firmness as the overall shape of the eyes change, often going from an youthful almond shape to a more round shape. In general, aged eyes give a tired appearance to the entire face.

5. D – An arching brow that rests above the upper eye bone socket and generally tapers to the outside of the face, leaving the peak at a 45-degree angle, best frames the eye. Men's eyebrows tend to be straight and somewhat flat. Totally thin or over plucked brows tend to be unflattering. Women's brows should begin thicker at the base — the area closer to the nose — and then taper outward to a thinner line.

6. True – And false! Gravity does appear to have some effect as it pulls facial tissue. One can see aging signs on the face of long-distance runners, where a more angular appearance, often perceived as more masculine, can develop. But is it gravity alone that causes signs of aging? The loss of facial fat makes the face more angular, which is why men are said to age better than women. Previously held theories that facial aging is attributed to *ptosis*, or drooping of the face *due to gravity alone*, is now disputed. Why? Gravity alone as a factor discounts the fact that the face covers multiple discrete anatomical regions. As such, the face may not age as a confluent mass.

7. **B** – A bit of a trick question, since profound sun damage, especially on a fair-skinned person, can cause significant premature aging. Other lifestyle and environmental factors, too, can age a person prematurely. Yet often to the outside world, it is the size and shape of a fuller mid face area that suggests a rested, more youthful appearance. The more volume there is in the mid face, the less sagging tissue there is. If the cheeks are prone to flatness, facial tissue sags downward, and this gives an appearance of being older. In extreme cases, a very thin face can appear haggard.

Micro Expressions

Because cosmetic surgery may involve a variety of very small alterations to achieve a meaningful rejuvenation, I want to briefly touch on micro expressions. In my practice, often the best results may eventually rest on a few tiny corrections, though the surgery itself may be extensive. For the most part, micro expressions are so fleeting we often don't notice them. That's why an apparently cheerful and friendly encounter with a stranger, buoyed with laughter and smiles, may give us pause as the stranger walks away. We think, "I'm not sure I trust him." Or a new employee smiles and responds cheerfully all day long, and yet we note a certain sadness underneath. Micro expressions are the reason why we instinctively have a different reaction to a situation when all outward signs *seem* to suggest one thing, but our gut tells us something else.

A micro expression (less than 1/25th of a second) is a fleeting and totally involuntary expression that no human being is able to hide. Most people are unable to identify micro expressions in themselves or others. Micro expressions surface when situations become risky and emotional stakes are raised, and the fleeting expressions cannot be controlled. A micro expression does not mean the person is necessarily dishonest and seeking to mislead another. High stakes for a painfully shy person could simply mean having to speak in front of a small group.

But the observant eye of a skilled surgeon will be able to isolate the micro expressions that make a person unique. The muscles in the face can adjust themselves into thousands of different configurations. There may be more than 10,000 possibilities. Could we really count them all and memorize each one? The point is that when eyes narrow just a fraction, or the corners of the mouth turn down a minuscule amount, this tiny change can produce an entirely different expression. It is up to the highly skilled surgeon to be able to make these micro adjustments in order to deliver beautiful results. Being able to read micro expressions helps a surgeon see beyond what may appear to be only a marginally different configuration. It is through these micro adjustments that your total expression, the one that makes you unique and beautiful, can change dramatically.

During a consultation, I am always looking for a patient's real smile. You may not be aware that all people use a "social smile," which is not a genuine smile. A social smile helps us navigate every day encounters with a certain ease. There's nothing wrong with a social smile. For the most part, it is not intended to be misleading. And if you've ever studied the smile of a losing Olympian as the gold medal is awarded to someone else, you can see that this social smile uses only the mouth muscles. The smiling loser puts on "a good face." But it is not a heartfelt, true smile. A true smile, known as a *Duchenne* smile, is quite distinctive. In the coming weeks, see if you can decipher the difference between a social smile and a real smile. In the latter, the eyes twinkle and narrow, causing the cheeks to rise. This is why I want to see the genuine smile in any patient consultation. After all, it's that rare and fleeting nuance that I must respect and protect in order to give each patient optimal results.

"Age is the acceptance of a term of years. But maturity is the glory of years"

— Martha Graham
American Dancer Choreographer

CHAPTER FOUR

How We Age

Nowadays, more men and women are adopting anti-aging strategies at a greater rate than previous generations did. The goal I most commonly hear from clients is, "I want to look as young as I feel!" Who can blame them? Adult Americans generally are healthier and more vital than their parents were at the same age. We've all heard it: Sixty is the new fifty, even the new forty. Also, since it's likely that today's workers will live longer, their desire to remain youthful — in both appearance and outlook — has other ramifications. For instance, people who love their professional pursuits are opting to work longer, past retirement age. Many launch a totally different new career, typically after their forties. Cosmetic enhancement was viewed strictly as a vanity concern a decade ago but it is now often seen to be a wise career choice. Earlier intervention, is more prevalent today. Rather than wait until their fifties, younger patients are exploring options, from fillers and Botox injections to facelift surgery. Those who opt for rejuvenation surgery at an earlier age typically take better care of their health and appearance following surgery. They're more aware of and vigilant about lifestyle choices and new strategies that prevent aging.

It is important to learn how best to protect the face and skin, and what measures you can take to better manage aging. Also, if you understand that the human face, even the most beautiful, is uneven or asymmetrical, it may help place some of your perceived shortcomings into perspective. This chapter is intended to help you ask better questions during your consultation. I hope it will help in developing an understanding of those decisions that drive a skilled surgeon's recommendations.

The Dynamics of Aging

A variety of interesting theories have been offered in an attempt to understand the dynamics of aging. Despite increased knowledge and research, however, a number of key questions and controversial issues still puzzle the experts. We know, for example, that our metabolic machinery — our gears, shock absorbers, and fuel-delivery system — gradually exhausts itself over time. The body, like any living thing, eventually wears out. Some experts suggest that cellular exhaustion results from the accumulation of oxidants and other destructive metabolic products. In other words, despite your having a clean and healthy lifestyle, something within your system may eventually go awry or break down. Genetics or hereditary factors are also key. We can't rearrange the DNA passed down by our forebears. Some scientists suggest that each cell is launched with a genetically programmed message. This cellular script guides the course of aging, practically predicting the time of each cell's natural death. Another explanation relates to genetic mutation known to occur during the growth and division of a cell. These may contribute to the aging process as well.

Lifestyle is a big factor, and it is something over which *you* can exert great control. Smoking, carrying too much weight, not getting enough sleep, avoiding regular exercise, excessive alcohol or drug use, and a poor diet will all increase signs of aging in a person. Environmental factors such as toxins, pollutants, or sun exposure also wreak havoc on our health and appearance. Whatever the cause, the result of aging skin is very much the same: The skin becomes thin, leathery, and wrinkled. Then, too, the complexion becomes dull and ashen. Conversely, youthful skin has three very specific attributes:

♦ Plumpness, accompanied by a moist, hydrated surface.

♦ Smooth, resilient cushioning beneath the skin,

♦ A vibrancy, regardless of race or skin color, that comes from healthy circulation.

The proverbial plump, dewy and colorful hands of an infant are an obvious example of these youthful traits.

Aging skin (noticeably of the neck, arms or hands) also shows an increase in uneven melanin production—the dark pigment that determines skin color. This may result in sporadic coloring; the most obvious signs are brown "liver spots." Finally, if you ever doubt the sun's ability to age you, examine a part of your body that is not exposed to the sun. The skin is far more plump and healthy looking, and that's why I urge you to wear sunblock and take other preventive measures.

Facial Aging Is Different

In addition to these broad changes in skin texture, the face has its own set of aging changes. In general, the plump, youthful fat layer beneath the skin diminishes. This fat loss, along with sun damage, compromises skin tone, and tissue support is generally weakened. If there is tooth loss, the jawline shrinks a bit. It's not all downhill, though, for some people. Certain features translate well as a person ages. For instance, a small, pert nose, sparkling eyes, or a natural upturned mouth with fuller lips can continue to impart a youthful look. But most of us, with average facial attributes, appear older when the following four, usually successive changes transpire:

❶ A hollow appearance in the cheeks. This results from fat, bone and soft tissue loss.

❷ A thinning of skin begins to spread to the temple area and around the upper eyelid.

❸ A general sagging of the face occurs.

❹ The envelope of facial skin does not shrink at the same rate as the skull; thus more sagging is obvious.

Skin wrinkles, another sign of aging, tend to cluster into three groups:

❶ Contour lines, the skin close to your earlobes or around the jawline, become less firm.

❷ Dynamic wrinkles, are caused by a contraction of facial muscles that are attached directly to the skin. Most are formed at right angles to the long axis where the muscle may contract or pull.

❸ "Gravity" lines, a function of our being upright creatures, are exaggerated over time by significant weight gain or loss or any stress that pulls at the attachments to the underlying facial tissue.

The face of a long-distance jogger often shows this wear and tear from gravity, environmental exposure, and also from extra fat loss. Certain serious ailments, such as diabetes, thyroid disorders, and Addison's disease or Cushing's disease (these stem from endocrine disorders), or chronic nutritional deficiencies will accelerate skin aging.

Other Changes That Come With Aging

Basic alterations in cellular structure — best studied under a microscope — contribute to aging. Yet the first signs of degeneration develop long before the human eye can see the signs. Characteristic changes occur in both layers of the skin: the epidermis, or upper layer, and the subcutaneous layer, the one beneath the skin.

In order to understand the changes below the surface, imagine the simple structure of a beautifully crafted couch, a valuable, antique hand-assembled centuries ago. When new, the fabric is taut, crisp and fresh, each pillow plump and yielding. Your epidermis is much like the upholstered outer fabric layer. Over time, it gradually becomes threadbare. The melanin-producing cells in the skin decrease, resulting in less protection against ultraviolet radiation. Like a well-worn feather cushion, resiliency is diminished.

The underlying dermis — this determines the thickness and texture of the skin — undergoes more significant changes during aging. Fibrous supporting tissue in this layer, composed of collagen fibers, the main structural protein of the body, thickens. Elastic fibers gradually deteriorate, contributing to a flaccid look. It's as if the furniture's supportive webbing and coils have lost their '*oomph.*' The couch is not sagging yet, but it has lost most of its supple cushioning power. When the subcutaneous fat becomes less thick, the fibrous connections with underlying tissue stretch a bit. Eventually there is loss of support. This is why skin eventually droops and sags.

How We Age: Decade by Decade.

Although facial sagging and wrinkling vary from person to person, the signs generally follow a characteristic cascade with each decade: from the forehead to the eyes to the nose and mouth to the chin and neck. Here's generally what happens with each decade:

◆ **Twenties** The first facial wrinkles are usually horizontal furrows in the forehead. Perhaps we frown a lot making our first important choices in life. Skin changes and damage may begin to accumulate below the surface, though most signs are not yet apparent. Your twenties could be considered "the age of prevention," when the skin should be protected vigilantly. A number of simple habits, each easily modified, can prevent aging. For instance, squinting in the sun and not using sunblock creates fine lines around the eyes. Too little sleep also ages a person. Drinking too much or smoking regularly dulls the complexion, and their collective stress on general health will take a considerable toll. Serious sunburn in the early years can set the stage for skin cancers of all types, including melanoma.

◆ **Thirties** First signs of laugh lines, and early indicators of crow's-feet appear. Sagging of upper lids (sometimes referred to as "hoods") begin to appear. There's a breakdown of the underlying skin-firming collagen and elastin; both lose structural strength. Skin becomes less elastic and loses its firm, supple texture. Sebaceous glands become less active, and skin dries out more frequently. Because poorly lubricated skin may not readily retain moisture, fine lines result.

◆ **Forties** Laugh lines deepen (perhaps we're happier now!) and skin on upper eyelids loses its smooth appearance, becoming increasingly redundant. Women's eye shadow begins to crease. A sharper line of demarcation between the lower eyelid and cheek begins to appear, producing a tired or wan look. The under-eye area may appear puffy. Lines that travel from the nose to the outside of the mouth (called nasolabial folds) become more obvious. Sagging skin over the jaw may form a jowl, and the crisp jaw line of youth often softens to a double chin. "Marionette lines" that run from the side of the mouth downward toward the chin may deepen.

◆ **Fifties** Cell turnover takes twice as long as it did at age 20. Thus, robust coloring and youthful radiance fade, and skin appears duller. The outside corners of the eyes begin to droop far more than before. Though patients often feel vibrant and cheery, the aging eye can yield a tired or sad appearance, further accentuated by a deepening of the nasolabial fold. More than any other decade, neck skin begins to sag and appear crepe-like. Stretched anterior neck muscles often contribute to the formation of bridle-like bands that travel vertically down the front of the neck. As these muscles continue to lose elasticity, a "turkey gobbler" may form. Some of this is due to weakening of the neck's platysma muscles on each side. As the underlying structure loses its strength, there is a natural thinning of the epidermis, which accelerates a papery skin appearance. Pigmentation becomes uneven, creating shadows, blotches, and dark circles under eyes; age spots appear on the face and the backs of the hands.

◆ **Sixties and older** The face is now mature, and the cushion of fat padding beneath the skin has diminished, leaving more angles and hollows. As muscle fibers weaken, some fat may remain under the eyes, forming bags. Facial bones may shrink, all-around sagging continues. The evidence of hormonal changes may lead to patchiness or unevenness in skin tone. The tip of the nose may droop a bit.

Some changes can be slowed, but specific facial exercises really won't do much to lift sagging features. Still, if you're willing to put in a little effort, some negative facial habits can be modified. Not all patients have great success, but others have learned to control excessive scowling or frowning. It may seem as if these expressions are involuntary, but they're not. Other patients opt for Botox. Finally, let's remember that several expressions are good for one's soul. Laughing and smiling rejuvenate the spirit. The more you laugh, the more able you are to elevate your mood. In other words, I hope you don't stop enjoying life just because you're afraid of a few lines!

Faces Are Asymmetrical

In truth, our bodies and faces tend to be asymmetrical and uneven. No matter your age, before considering surgery understand that all faces tend to be a bit *off*. And it's wise to quantify how asymmetrical your features are, since as you heal, you'll scrutinize your anatomy as you have never done before. A number of patients begin to notice things that they're convinced are new developments following surgery. And perhaps you'll be tempted to blame a skilled surgeon for tampering with your alleged symmetry. What's the best way to assess facial symmetry?

One of the better tests is easy. Simply stand in front of a mirror and tip your head back. Imagine a coin is balanced on the tip of your nose. Continue to tip your head backward as you try to read the underside of the coin. Now hold that pose. See how your features "fall" across your face. You may notice one eye is noticeably larger, perhaps wider than the other. Your nostrils may flare in an uneven fashion. Or perhaps they flare evenly but the nose seems to tip slightly to one side. Your ears may not line up evenly, or the right side of your jaw may not the match the left side. The purpose of this simple test is not to make you feel bad. The real goal is for us to accept that asymmetry exists. Sure, you may wish to fix some attributes. But I also hope you will be able to embrace imperfections as part of being human. We all wish to look as good as we possibly can look. But if you strive for perfection at all costs, you may be setting yourself up for a string of disappointments.

Profiles are another way to evaluate symmetry. For instance, a receding chin makes practically any nose appear too small or too large. In general, even "perfect" features are thrown out of proportion by certain facial structures that somehow attract unwanted attention. The degree to which the eye is distracted often defines imperfections, much the way that we note a tiny scratch on the door of a shiny new sports car. In sum, we all have a variety of facial imperfections. Rather than despair, it's wise to determine which ones cause you concern and discuss remedies with a skilled surgeon.

What Is Beauty, Anyway?

So what makes a face beautiful? Clearly, muscles play a significant role. Bone structure, too, is critically important. But there are other considerations. We've heard that "beauty is in the eye of the beholder." That's certainly true. What one person finds attractive, another might find less than perfect or merely odd.

Unfortunately, some people focus negatively on a perfectly normal attribute — unnoticeable to others — and fixate about its shortcomings. For instance, early in her career, Marilyn Monroe was advised by a casting agent that the space between her nose and her lip was too short. Too short? She fretted about this "imperfection" for most of her career. I offer this as an example of how silly and dangerous certain beauty guidelines and imagined shortcomings can be.

When considering facial beauty, let me offer some structural basics that help us understand why some attributes are valued and others are not. Much has to do with proportion. Basically, the overriding shape of the face tends to be oval, like an egg. Some real-life variations on the oval ideal include:

◆ Triangular (the forehead is broader than the chin, which is pointed)

◆ Square

◆ Round

The face falls into three basic parts. The first third is from the hairline to the upper eyelids. The next third is the upper lids to the base of the nostrils. Finally, from the nostrils down to the chin creates the remaining third segment, of which the neck, too, is often considered to be an integral part. Each of these is addressed in separate chapters 5, 6 and 7.

Beyond these basics, there are some generally accepted standards that our American society, for better or for worse, feels contribute to a person's general attractiveness. These include:

◆ The upper lip should be full in a 1:2 ratio to the lower lip. In general, narrow, thin lips are associated with aging and are considered to be less appealing than fuller, more robust lips.

◆ The nose is a personal preference, though Americans seem to favor what I call a "generic" nose. One hardly notices a generic nose. Europeans, on the whole, show more acceptance, even preference, for a wide variety of noses. There, a magnificent profile, one where the nose is almost remarkable, can be seen as a prized possession. It's as if a person's individual character is displayed via a profile. In the U.S., a desired nasal tip is thin and almost delicate, forming an equilateral triangle when viewed from the base. The nostrils are equal in size and oval-shaped.

◆ Eyes are the most expressive facial trait. Generally, they are separated by the "average" length of one eye, though some of our revered American beauties, Jackie Kennedy Onassis being an example, are exceptions. We prefer eye placement that is mostly symmetrical. Beautiful eyes lack sagging upper lids, which may convey a sad or tired look.

- Ears rest against the head in a generally flat manner, with the base of each lobe about even with the nostril line.

- The chin, viewed sideways, creates an approximate 90-degree angle with the neck. Ideally, the chin creates facial harmony and generally lines up with an imaginary line dropped perpendicular to the border of the lower lip.

Quick Review

- If you understand the basics of aging, you may better understand what your surgeon can and cannot do. Facelifts by a skilled surgeon can produce remarkable and beautiful results. But cosmetic surgery to reduce signs of aging rarely produces miracles.

- Most beautiful faces and bodies are uneven. We're, asymmetrical and that's part of being human.

- The rules of proportion are general guidelines; they are best applied judiciously.

- Be flexible when assessing what you want fixed. Be aware there are simply some things cosmetic surgery cannot remedy.

- The condition of a person's skin plays a pivotal role in cosmetic surgery. 🦐

"If wrinkles must be written on our brow, let them not be written on our heart. The spirit should never grow old"

— James A. Garfield
20th President of the United States

CHAPTER FIVE

The Upper Face:

Superior Rejuvenation

For the average person, often the brow area or forehead show early signs of aging. The reason for this is simple: the upper portion of the face is one of the more emotionally expressive areas. We use it a lot. Many of us habitually furrow our brow when puzzled. We raise our eyebrows when surprised. It's difficult to show concern without some brow movement. Over time, lines, creases and deep furrows develop and as they appear, they impart an impression of anxiety, anger or apprehension. When a brow begins to droop, it makes a person appear sad or tired, though your actual demeanor may be energized and bright. These signs become more pronounced through the years, primarily due to muscle movement, though heredity may play a role.

Innovative Brow Treatments

Fortunately, there are a variety of cosmetic options today to restore a more youthful appearance to the brow. These range from injections to lasers as well as surgery — or a combination of two or three treatments. For instance, Botox or Dysport which are injections to block signals to muscles from nerves, are often used in conjunction with fillers to reduce fine lines. Sun damage is the exception to this approach: neither

Botox, Dysport and/or fillers will diminish sun damage aging. For reformed sun worshipers, laser treatment is the best therapy. Lasers also treat a myriad of other skin imperfections that may detract from a more youthful look. Nonetheless, when a brow is marred by more advanced aging, surgery tends to be the best remedy. A browlift, also called a forehead lift, corrects a sagging brow and smooths forehead furrows. With some patients, browlifts alone may improve the arch of the eyebrow and somewhat rejuvenate the eyes, though the surgery is typically performed in conjunction with eye rejuvenation procedures.

Often patients are uncertain if a browlift will give them the refreshed look they desire. To help clarify the signs of forehead aging, generally lines and brow furrows tend to cluster in three types of formations, which become increasingly visible, over time. These, illustrated in the drawing Figure 5-1, include:

◆ forehead lines

◆ glabellar creases (known informally as number 11s)

◆ general drooping of the brow itself

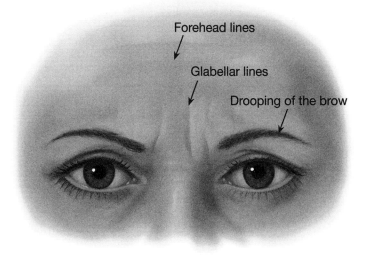

Figure 5-1

Furrows that appear deeply "etched" occur when the support network of collagen and elastin breaks down. As the skin loses its support structure, elasticity diminishes and the area becomes lax. Eventually, layers of muscle weaken and the 'cushions' of fat that cover underlying bone are depleted.

Benefits of Brow Treatments

Cosmetic procedures to treat the brow area vary according to the signs of aging and a patient's individual needs, though generally, corrective procedures are designed to achieve the following goals: diminish forehead frown lines and the creases between the eyebrows, raise eyebrows to a more youthful and engaged position, minimize expression lines that occur above the bridge of the nose.

If you're contemplating a more youthful brow, discuss your expectations with a skilled and qualified surgeon. For instance, if you don't mind a few forehead lines but wish to lose the omnipresent scowl, perhaps Botox or Dysport injections are what you'll need. If your eyebrows and brow area droop, surgery may be the best option.

This chapter offers insight about the most effective treatments to rejuvenate and refresh your brow area. To assess your specific needs, stand in front of a mirror and close your eyes. Relax your forehead. Allow all tension and expression to simply evaporate. Slowly open your eyes. What does your brow reveal? Do you see horizontal forehead lines?

Is it difficult to discern your upper eyelids because your brow droops over it? Do you have deep, permanent vertical lines — they look like the number '11'— in the space between your eyebrows? Do these lines make you look concerned, even grouchy? Have you lost the beautiful curve of a youthful brow that frames your eyes?

These particular concerns may indicate that a brow rejuvenation will help ameliorate your individual signs of aging.

How To Treat Some Aging Signs

Botox or Dysport Injections

When lines are fine — appearing to be superficial rather than deep grooves — the treatment is simpler. With minor signs of aging, injections that immobilize muscles may be your first line of defense. Botox or Dysport works by blocking signals from the nerves to those muscles that contract and create wrinkles. In essence, the 'offending' muscle is simply paralyzed and stays in a relaxed mode. Specific muscles can be targeted. One prominent area is the glabella region, the area between the eyebrows. Other forehead wrinkles, known as dynamic wrinkles since they are caused by muscle contractions, can be treated as well, though it's worth repeating: Creases and wrinkles from sun damage (called static wrinkles because they remain after muscle relaxation) do not respond.

Typically, multiple areas are addressed in one session and the average treatment only takes minutes using a fine needle. Most patients experience little pain, and an ice pack afterward can minimize minor discomfort. Depending on the patient and the expertise of the doctor, minor bruising may appear — or not. If you are pregnant, breastfeeding or have certain neurological diseases, clearly you should not use Botox or Dysport.

A more relaxed expression will materialize within one or two days, though the desired full effect may take up to ten days. In general, results vary by person, but most patients experience meaningful benefits that last up to four months. As the effect wears off, lines gradually reappear. For some patients, a series of successive injections extended over longer time periods tends to lessen the reappearance of wrinkles and some patients report longer lasting effects.

Fillers.

Like Botox or Dysport, soft tissue fillers are another first line defense in the treatment of aging skin. While the optimal age for filler patients used to be in those in their 40s to early 50s, I see more patients in their mid 30s each year. On the plus side, fillers can dramatically alter the early signs of aging In fact, younger patients who choose fillers seem to postpone the signs of the aging process more effectively. How so? It seems that "early adopters" are simply more dedicated to leading anti aging lifestyles. They consistently use sunscreen. They adopt a regular and better at home skin care regimen; they value a healthy diet, one that is rich in antioxidants and minerals. They drink plenty of water, avoid excessive alcohol, don't smoke, get enough sleep and regularly exercise.

Still, fillers should not be taken lightly. In the wrong hands, unsightly results, including unnatural and irregular contour problems, even lumps, can develop. Since fillers work best under the skin to replace elasticity and to plump skin, the ideal candidate is someone who has started to have some volume loss with lines around the mouth. Additionally, there may be some hollowness in the cheek area. From an aesthetic perspective, plumping in these areas can have a wonderful outcome and take years off. But if there's pronounced sagging, fillers are not an effective option. This is the main pitfall of what is commonly known as "the liquid facelift." A procedure with a cute name meant to fulfill the fantasy that true facelift results can be achieved with fillers and the occasional strategically placed Botox or Dysport injection. I find that many practices promote the "liquid facelift" as a unique procedure but it's not. It's just another way to creatively market fillers to plump up deep furrows. Practices that push the liquid option as a "lift" typically are practices that don't perform surgery; some even try to capitalize on fears of surgery. However, the plain truth is that advanced aging, in most instances, is best treated via surgery.

The downside to fillers is that they are not a permanent solution; on average, they last from a few months to a year, though some patients enjoy benefits that do extend beyond a year. And despite their "touch up" reputation, it may be best to avoid a "lunch time" quick visit your first time. That's because with any injection there may be some redness, swelling and even bruising. If you plan to return to work that same day, you may be fine, perhaps no one will notice or ask questions. But it's possible, like some patients who are more sensitive, that mild temporary swelling or redness may make you self-conscious.

What are the more popular filler brands? Radiesse, Juvederm, Restylane, Perlane, Captique and Prevelle Silk are made of hyaluronic acid, a naturally occurring substance found in the body that is essential to plump and youthful-looking skin. I believe these non animal source hyaluronic acids deliver a smoother, more natural appearance. And since the body already produces this chemical naturally, allergic reaction is very rare. Before the introduction of today's fillers, most dermal injections used animal products such as bovine collagen (derived from cows), silicone (sometimes toxic), or a person's own body fat. Since each filler type has a slightly different consistency, you must have confidence that your doctor understands how to select the right filler and how deep to inject it. Before agreeing to treatment, please seriously confirm that his or her expertise in this area stems from solid experience over time and across a wide variety of patients. Also, consistency may dictate which filler is best suited to treat a particular area, so remain open to which option may work best for you. In other words, don't request a particular brand; listen to what your skilled surgeon suggests.

Like all cosmetic procedures, your results may vary from those of your friends or even from the norm. There are many variables such as skin texture, age, sun damage, smoking, lifestyle history, genetics, and metabolic factors. These all are likely to influence your outcome. And your doctor's preferences and skill with injecting fillers will directly impact results. In sum, the filler that works best for each patient is best judged on a case-by-case basis. Finally, one important tip: Be candid during your consultation about what medicines you take, including vitamins and supplements. I recommend patients eliminate aspirin, ibuprofen, and vitamin E at least five days before a scheduled filler procedure. This simple precaution appears to minimize bruising.

Other Brow Options

There are several other treatments typically used in conjunction with brow rejuvenation. Each offers distinctive benefits for achieving a smoother and more youthful brow. Some of the more effective approaches I use include the following.

Lasers

Lasers offer effective skin treatments and many cosmetic surgeons rely on them to treat various aesthetic issues. To help understand laser efficacy — there are dozens of brand names and despite lots of information, patients remain confused — this quick summary may help you understand how lasers work. "LASER" is actually an acronym which stands for "Light Amplification by the Stimulated Emission of Radiation." In simple terms, lasers are concentrated forms of light with specific wavelengths that are absorbed by specific pigments called chromophores.

In cosmetic procedures, laser treatments are adjusted by the wavelength, the size of the area to be treated and the duration of treatment. Laser treatments should be chosen according to the aesthetic goal of your desired outcome. Be clear about what you would like to change and improve about your skin's appearance.

In my experience, lighter toned people have two major concerns. The first concern relates to superficial wrinkling and discoloration; these tend to stem from aging and sun exposure. The second concern relates to broken capillaries and uneven skin tones due to accumulated sun exposure. Fortunately, lasers can be used to treat superficial layers as well as the deeper layers of the skin. My approach is to start by treating the deeper layers of the skin first, particularly uneven skin tones which are most visible to patients. After the underlying problems have been treated, the next step is to identify the best type of superficial treatment. Within the realm of superficial treatments, there are several options including gentle chemical peels, microdermabrasion and topical laser treatments. The great thing about treating deeper layers first, followed by superficial treatments, is that once you have completed the first stage, the patient may require less in the topical, more superficial treatment stage.

Microfractional CO_2 Laser

This particular instrument is a truly innovative anti aging breakthrough, one that really has revolutionized rejuvenation strategies for a wide array of patient types. The microfractional CO_2 laser utilizes the effectiveness of traditional carbon dioxide lasers — these remain the gold standard in wrinkle removal — without some of the harsh side effects. The microfractional CO_2 laser deploys an improved application technique that essentially delivers powerful results without the traditional complications that plagued other lasers. In other words, the patient derives all the benefits of laser resurfacing, which is still the best way to remove wrinkles, with less downtime and without the painful consequences.

In layman terms, without becoming too technical, microfractional CO_2 laser therapy delivers a precise matrix of micro spots that penetrate the skin. This penetration stimulates the formation of new collagen. At the same time, there's immediate shrinking of damaged tissue. The methodology results in a faster healing process with less pain. Many types of microfractional CO_2 laser, including the one I use, will generally require only one treatment in most cases.

The improvements are visible in three areas. First, there's immediate tightening with the contraction of collagen fibers and this reduces wrinkles. Loose skin is noticeably improved. Second, textural irregularities are diminished or removed. These include pigmentation problems, enlarged pores and acne scars. Third, sun damage and aging discoloration as well as certain skin lesions such as actinic keratoses can be effectively addressed. Patients love the microfractional CO_2 Laser therapy because it speeds the healing process, enabling them to return to their normal daily routines in less down time.

IPL

Intense pulsed light, known as IPL Photo rejuvenation, is another tool to refine and beautify the brow area, though it works on other parts of the body such as décolleté, arms, legs and hands. IPL is a safe, non-invasive skin treatment that diminishes signs of aging, especially those due to sun damage. The technique allows highly controlled light and heat to penetrate the layers of the skin. This stimulates the growth of new collagen, while treating excess pigment, redness, spider veins, fine lines and enlarged pores. Benefits include a more even skin tone, smoother skin, lessening of fine wrinkles and sun damage.

A cold gel is applied to the treatment area and treatments are fairly easy on the patient, without much discomfort, if any. A session lasts about 20 minutes and generally a series of 4 to 6 six sessions is recommended for optimal results. Normal activities can begin immediately after treatment. Some patients experience slight swelling, redness, or even a darkening of brown spots in the treatment area immediately afterwards but these are likely to fade or disappear completely within 24 hours. Ice can be used to diminish any swelling.

Are You A Candidate for Brow Surgery?

A forehead lift, or browlift, elevates the soft tissue and skin of the forehead and brow Surgery can help raise the brow line higher and reduce the appearance of lines and wrinkles, restoring a firmer, more youthful appearance to the upper portion of the face. The procedure tightens loose skin, minimizes or removes forehead wrinkles, and corrects a certain amount of drooping in the eye area. The surgery is an effective means to rejuvenate one's appearance and return focus to the beauty of the eye area.

Both men and women can benefit from browlift rejuvenation. Since men tend to have heavier brows than women, a female drooping brow may imbue a somewhat masculine appearance. Conversely, a beautifully arched eyebrow is a sign of youth; it tends to dramatize the eye area. That's why many women pluck brows, seeking to restore a youthful, more feminine arch. For some women, it is important to have a high "upper eyelid and brow platform"— which means that the upper lid and brow areas are elevated; there are no excess creases to hide eye shadow, for instance. Eye makeup is able to create the illusion the woman desires. If a woman enjoyed naturally arched eyebrows in her youth, then this is a look to restore. Conversely, women who have had naturally level brows would look perpetually surprised and artificial with the wrong browlift. A man's overdone browlift, which may result in a brow that is too high or too arched, also may yield an unnatural and disappointing result. As with all cosmetic procedures, browlifts should be customized to the individual in order to impart a natural youthful appearance.

For all cosmetic surgeries, final results will vary from patient to patient. In general, I perform these types of lifts as an outpatient procedure under local anesthesia with intravenous sedation for comfort. The surgery averages from one to two hours. Since a browlift can significantly reduce the frown lines between the eyes, it is frequently performed in conjunction with upper and/or lower eyelid surgery as well as with facelift surgery. In my opinion, this combination delivers optimal results.

Endoscopic Lift

Years ago, forehead surgery generally involved a procedure known as the coronal lift. It required a long incision, typically spanning from ear to ear, over the top of the head. Thankfully, we now have a more innovative approach. The endoscopic lift requires less recovery time and deploys a minimal incision. With endoscopic surgery, the surgeon makes several small incisions, perhaps four to six, within a person's hairline. They can be as short as half an inch, and some incisions may be slightly longer. A tiny camera, about the size of a pencil's eraser tip, is inserted under the skin so that the surgeon can survey muscles responsible for creating the deep furrows and surrounding tissue. During surgery, the treated muscles and tissue are secured; skin is shifted backward to a more youthful repose and sutured closed.

With a browlift, there may be minor swelling and bruising around the forehead, cheeks and eyes. Finally, for a browlift to appear completely natural, the resulting expression must be harmonious. If the arch is artificial, a person appears caught off guard and perpetually surprised. When the inner half of a brow is raised at the expense of the outer brow, a sad expression often results. The best way to prevent these unfortunate results is through selection of a qualified and highly experienced cosmetic surgeon. In sum: make your consultation a productive session by getting clear answers to all of your questions — have them prepared ahead of time — and by speaking with several recent patients.

The Trichophytic Browlift

Hair loss may be an undesirable result of a brow lift when the incision permanently destroys hair roots. Unfortunately, most surgeons simply avoid discussing this issue or raising this possibility. In part this may be traceable to how surgeons generally survey a patient's face. Many tend to focus on skin surface and features alone. Rarely do they step back and study the ramifications beyond the hairline. Some — even a few of the big name 'society' surgeons — are not trained in the newer, more innovative incisions that permit healthy hair re-growth. They have developed their single, individual approach and have built a reputation by doing lifts their way. Others are reluctant to change or adapt.

Before agreeing to surgery, understand that a brow lift, in some cases, may actually accelerate the appearance of aging. This occurs when unexpected hair thinning results via a misplaced incision or due to an elevated hairline, one that lengthens the area of the forehead. A wise and highly skilled surgeon will

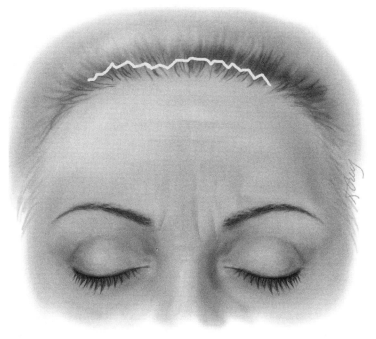

Figure 5-2

evaluate each patient in order to effectively screen those who may genetically be at risk for hair loss or who may look older with a larger forehead.

To minimize hair attrition, a different incision may permit hair to grow through the scar, making it difficult to see an incision, even with a short haircut. This innovative "in the hairline" approach is one I prefer and the results have been excellent. The incision creates a somewhat irregular line, a sort of zig-zag, rather than a straight cut. Technically known as the trichophytic closure or incision, it is placed just behind the hairline and is done only under the skin — as opposed to the deep tissue placement, like various older browlift techniques.

Personally, I view this technique to be the superior option for the right candidate and the results endure over time, delivering a more meaningful benefit to my patients. Do some research, ask good sources you may know to see if you can locate a surgeon who is experienced in the benefits of this particular technique.

Quick Review

♦ Be clear about possible results via a thorough consultation with your surgeon. Match expectations with a realistic outcome.

♦ Subtle signs of aging may be best treated via Botox or Dysport injections as well as fillers or other non invasive approaches.

♦ Persons with pronounced brow drooping see more meaningful results via surgery.

♦ Nearly all surgery patients will see improvement in horizontal lines.

♦ Most forehead surgery will diminish some lateral 'hooding' over the upper eyelid. However, significant or pronounced eye aging is best treated by separate eye and face rejuvenation procedures.

♦ Nearly any hairline surgery offers the potential to disrupt future hair growth. Be sure your surgeon does not discount the potential for hair loss. Ask how any incision may compromise future hair growth, no matter how thick your hair is today! 🖝

"Beauty is how you feel inside, and it reflects in your eyes. It is not something physical."

— Sophia Loren
Film Star

CHAPTER SIX

Eye Rejuvenation

Our eyes are among the most important facial features, so when tissues in this area begins to age, our overall appearance is affected. The process of aging eyes is gradual. It happens with nearly every blink of an eye. A *blink* of an eye? Can that be true?

The analogy is not much of an exaggeration. The eye area is delicate, the skin is especially thin, and eventually, as the support structure becomes lax, aging signs appear. At first there may be only fine lines; later, a bit of drooping and sagging; and finally bags, commonly called puffy eyes, appear. Puffy eyes linger even after a solid night of sleep. Since the increments of aging accrue slowly, often *we* are not the first to notice. Women who wear makeup tend to be more aware, especially when the perfect cream foundation begins to crease. As one patient lamented, "All of a sudden that expensive concealer doesn't seem to hide much of anything anymore!"

Since puffy eyes convey a look that suggests, "I'm overworked," or "I didn't get enough sleep last night," coworkers may first raise your awareness. They wonder if you're feeling okay. That's why new patients may express their frustration. They feel great! But their friends, family, and colleagues remark on how tired they look.

Eyelid surgery, also known as **blepharoplasty**, improves the appearance of the upper eyelids, lower eyelids, or both. The surgery is designed to impart a rejuvenated appearance so that you look more rested and alert.

In this chapter, I'll describe several of the more innovative ways to refresh and rejuvenate the eyes. There are both surgical and nonsurgical procedures. Some patients may benefit from a single approach or a combination of several. When appropriate, I'll describe how my technique offers a meaningful point of difference from other procedures. As you read, you may wonder, "Do I even need *any* work?" Or "Am I a candidate?" "What's the right age for eye surgery?" "What are the risks?"

Aesthetics and Delicacy

Over the years, I've observed many cosmetic surgeons who seem to regard eyelifts as almost an afterthought. These surgeons are comfortable with older-style surgeries. To them, eyelift surgery is an aesthetic postscript. But an eyelift can't possibly be reduced to a simple nip and tuck. I'd like to explain why.

During my training as an eye microsurgeon, I witnessed the intricacies of the eye's structure. The wonders of the human eye and the elaborate interwoven network of the surrounding anatomy are astonishing. That's why eyelid complexity and delicacy demand an exceptionally high level of skill.

A top cosmetic surgeon's expertise is inextricably linked to *artistic discretion*. In the end, once structural integrity has been achieved, eyelid surgery is really about *aesthetics*. Without the skilled expertise of an aesthetic specialist, a slightly imprecise surgical decision can dramatically alter any person's characteristic look. In reality, the best cosmetic eye surgeons are artists who instinctively execute a myriad of micro adjustments that cumulatively deliver a quantum result to the patient. These micro adjustments delivered by virtue of a high level of skill are nevertheless governed by an aesthetic sensibility. Eyelifts are no simple nip and tucks!

As a specialist, there are times when I am called upon to correct the work of other surgeons. In some cases, the previous result actually aged the patient. In other cases, the patient's eyelids were unable to close. The eyelids and the surrounding skin and muscles that control them convey our emotions. This delicate network must support any correction the surgeon makes. If the skin and underlying structure are not treated with absolute skill and precision, you may be trading aging signs for a distracting asymmetrical outcome or a distortion that may require additional corrective means.

In sum, that's why eyelift surgery cannot be an easy one-size-fits-all procedure. Each procedure is remarkably different for every right eye and left eye and from patient to patient. The surrounding area must maintain an intimate and inextricable relationship with the eye.

Eye Aging Is Different

Every blink we experience causes the tiniest stretch of elastic fibers in the skin. Blinking also stretches fibers of the eyelid's *levator* muscle, the one that raises the eyelid. As the area's thinner skin begins to show fine lines, the overall underlying structure also ages. It begins to sag and droop as the muscle layers weaken. Volume in our younger years normally gives eyelids a full and supple appearance. However, this youthful volume, a form of fat, is depleted over time. Fatty deposits around the eye that remain may eventually shift in response to weakened, sagging muscles. This shift results in puffiness and can create bags around the eyes. All of these aging signs make a person appear weary, even sad. For many, the turning point arrives when they are viewed to be older than their actual years. Genetic factors can contribute to premature aging signs. Many young adults are dismayed that bags — just like Granddad's — materialize well before their middle age.

Patients frequently ask me to identify the best age for an eyelift. Is it thirty-five years of age? Or forty? Based on my practice, I can say with certainty *there is no ideal age.* The need for eye rejuvenation varies widely, across several decades. I've worked on many patients in their twenties. Some inherited a hollowed and wan look that belied their youth. Others, in their early thirties, had bags and hooded upper lids. And I've worked on patients well into their eighties and nineties.

There is an increase in one demographic group, however. Today's high-powered executives want to look vibrant and energized. After all, their careers are thriving. Why shouldn't they appear equally robust? As one banker suggested, "I can't afford to look as if I stayed up all night to get the PowerPoint presentation done!" Her message was clear: looking refreshed imparts an alert sensibility. And yes, a refreshed appearance can help forge a healthy competitive edge. This perspective is borne out by national statistics. According to the American Society for Aesthetic Plastic Surgery, *eyelifts have become the most sought-after cosmetic facial surgery procedure,* surpassing the facelift, rhinoplasty, facial implants, and forehead lifts.

If you're "starting over" with a new career or getting back into the dating scene, it's common to become more self-conscious about your looks and any age-related changes you see. Major events such as weddings motivate others to seek cosmetic eyelid surgery. No matter your age or motivation, here's what you need to know.

Architecture of the Eye Area

Before we tackle how eyelid surgery works, understanding the underlying structure can help clarify which approach may work *best for you*. Like the rest of the face, the eyelids are composed of soft tissue that contain layers of skin and muscle. Behind the soft tissue, there's orbital fat, which gives shape to the eyes and other tissues in the orbit, the space in the skull where the eyeball sits. In order to be a good candidate for a blepharoplasty, a patient must have sufficient surrounding structures to support the procedure.

Each eye has two lids; the upper lid acts like a windshield wiper, and when closed, the lids distribute tears over the surface of the eye. Ideally, both upper lids are similar, but this could change with age. There are a number of muscles, too. The key ones include the *orbicularis* muscle, which closes the eye, and the previously mentioned *levator* muscle, which raises the upper lid. The other muscles that move each eyeball are not particularly pertinent to eyelid surgery, except for one of the smallest. The *inferior oblique* muscle may be encountered

"Though we travel the world over to find the beautiful, we must carry it with us or we find it not"

— Ralph Waldo Emerson

American author, poet and philosopher

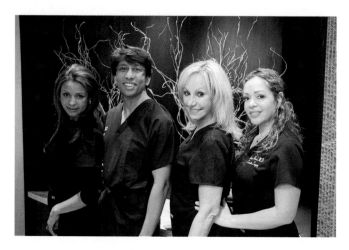

"The staff at Dr. Prasad's office treated me like one of the family. As a nurse in a hospital, I know how busy a surgical suite can be. I felt very comfortable with the level of attention I received, and I recommend them without reservation."

—Susan K., Registered Nurse

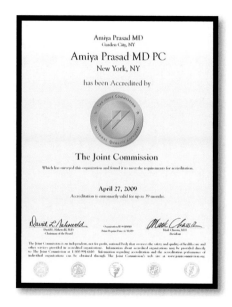

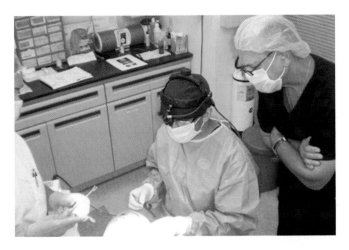

Surgeons from all over the world come to study Dr. Prasad's techniques in Facial Cosmetic Procedures.

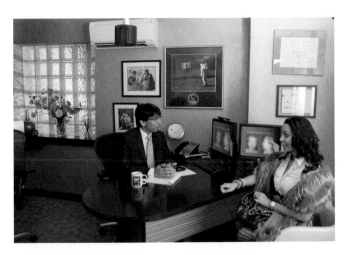

"I chose Dr. Prasad as my surgeon because he spent a lot of time with me and really understood my concerns. He is a very good listener, which I found was unique compared to other consultations that I have had."   — *Amy S., Magazine Editor*

Sharing the Experience

For many of our clients, looking younger restores both their appearance and their confidence. We often hear phrases like "After the procedure, I look on the outside, the way I feel on the inside!" They often share their stories by writing testimonials and appearing on news programs.

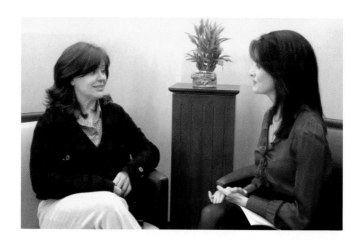

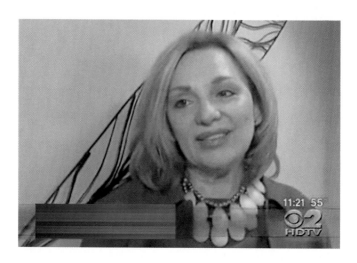

Non Surgical Facial Rejuvenation

There are several new technologies and non surgical treatments which can help people look their best. The challenge for the consumer is to find the right treatments provided by highly qualified specialists. In our practice, non surgical treatments help address the areas which are ususally not addressed by surgery and are part of a treatment system to help people look their best.

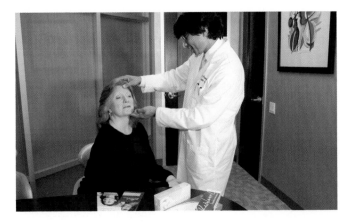

Dr. Prasad is using Pellevé™, a radio-frequency based non-surgical skin tightening procedure to help improve fine lines and tighten loose skin.

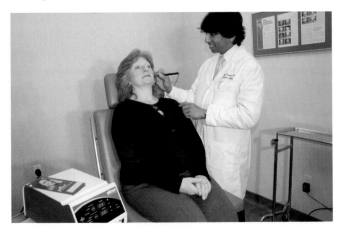

> Every face is unique and has a distinctive character
> which gives it a "je ne sais quoi". Aesthetic Rejuvenation
> is about preserving this feature while balancing how you feel
> on the inside with how you *look* on the outside.
>
> — Amiya Prasad, M.D., F.A.C.S.

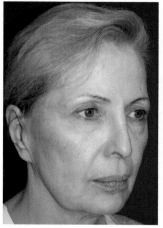 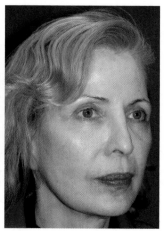

Before   After

This 62 year-old international marketing firm head became aware that she was perceived as "too old" for a project after overhearing some unkind remarks about her appearance during a presentation. She is a truly dynamic and highly energetic woman, which was not being communicated by her face. We performed rejuvenation surgery for her eyes and face. Since her procedure, she has not faced any "age" discrimination. She was so moved by her experience that she created her own photographic diary of her experience and made a PDF which is downloadable at our website.

To say that the eyes are the windows to the soul means more today than ever. We judge intention, sincerity, trustworthiness, confidence and form all sorts of opinions based on the look we see in someone's eyes. The appearance of tired-looking eyes affects how others perceive you and can significantly affect your social life and your career.

Eye rejuvenation surgery has to preserve the language that you telegraph with your eyes, so it needs to be done just right. We see too many examples of eyes which appear "overdone" after cosmetic surgery. Employing advanced techniques with an artistic eye is the key to natural eye rejuvenation.

— Amiya Prasad, M.D., F.A.C.S.

Upper and Lower Eyelift

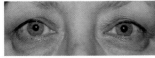 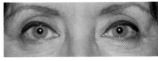

Before   After

Restoring a brighter and natural appearance to the eyes are the main concerns for women who come for eye rejuvenation procedures.

Lower Eyelid Lift

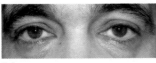 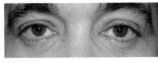

Before   After

People are surprised to learn that **50%** of our clients for eyelid rejuvenation are men. Maintaining a masculine quality during the rejuvenation procedure is an art in itself. Too many celebrities exhibit the telltale signs of surgery. For this reason, many of our male clients do extensive research before electing to have their procedure with us. We routinely show before and after photos of our patients to give prospective clients a feel for our unique approach.

135

Ethnic Considerations

As communication makes the world seem closer, many now refer to the world as "flat". New definitions of aesthetic beauty result from the blending of many ethnicities and are reflected in fashion and entertainment daily. Understanding the unique characteristics of eyes of all ethnicities has been a distinction that I have been proud to demonstrate in my practice. It is a priority when I teach cosmetic eyelid rejuvenation to colleagues.

— Amiya Prasad, M.D., F.A.C.S.

Upper and Lower Eyelift

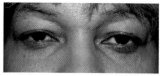
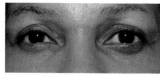

Before

After

Restoring a brighter and natural appearance to the eyes are the main concerns for women who come for eye rejuvenation procedures.

Lower Eyelid Lift

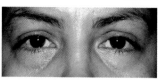
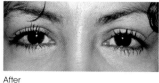

Before

After

These two women had specific concerns about recovering the youthful appearance of their eyes, but they wanted to maintain the individual appearance and shape of the eyes that is seen in African-American and Hispanic women respectively. We were able to preserve the balance of their eyes, nose and mouth to the width of their face, in which both were both quite pleased with the results.

Ethnic Considerations

People of Asian origin have visited our office from all over
the world for the "double eyelid" crease. They seek naturally
appearing lid creases, which is a well-accepted sign
of attractiveness. They don't want to have eyes that appear
"Europeanized". The key is to perform the procedure
so that the eyelids resemble the Asian eyes of those
who were born with lid creases. The people who seek out
our services are relieved that we appreciate
the importance of the lid crease, and we understand how
to achieve the culturally desirable appearance.

— *Amiya Prasad, M.D., F.A.C.S.*

Creating a "Double Eyelid"

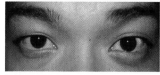 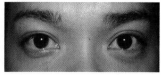

Before   After

This young 25 year-old man had been saving up to get the
desired eyelid creases. He had partial creases that he felt
were a distraction from his appearance, and he felt that we
understood the subtlety of the look he was seeking.

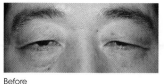 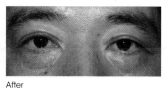

Before   After

This 55 year-old man had been bothered by his lack of creases
for years but chose not to do anything about it. That was until
his signs of aging caught up with him, and his eyelids actually
interfered with his vision. He had lid creases and an upper eyelid lift done to improve his vision. He was not bothered by the
lower lid bags that he had. He felt that they were appropriate
for his appearance so he elected to leave them alone.

PTOSIS

Ptosis (pronounced toe-sis) is frequently seen in people considering eyelid rejuvenation particularly after the age of 60. Failure to recognize the presence of ptosis is the source of disappointment for many people who have upper eyelid surgery. The most common reason for the eyes to droop is a muscle called the "levator" (like "elevator"), which is responsible for lifting the eyelid. It can be seen in younger people since it is sometimes congenital. It is commonly caused by thinning of the muscle tissue leading the eyes to droop. Surgical correction of ptosis is technically advanced and requires years of experience. I use an analogy about correction of ptosis compared with routine upper eyelid surgery.

I say it's like piloting a plane compared to driving a car.

Upper and Lower Eyelift with Correction of Upper Eyelid Ptosis (drooping of the upper eyelids from thinning of the muscle which lifts the eyelids)

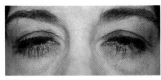
Before

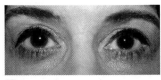
After

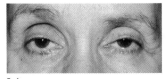
Before

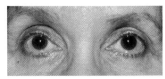
After

COMPLICATIONS

Approximately 20% of my practice is related to performing revision surgery for eyelids and facelifts. People have traveled from all over the U.S. and the world for our services.

All surgeons experience complications; however, with expertise and depth of experience, many of them can be avoided.

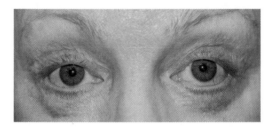

This is an example of a patient who traveled from somewhere in the United States for complications from cosmetic facial surgery. This woman had three surgeries prior to coming to us for Aesthetic Reconstructive Surgery of the lower eyelids. She required skin grafting and special materials to the front and back of the lower eyelids.

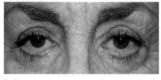
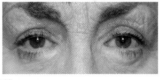

Before   After

This 63 year-old woman had eyelid surgery performed by another surgeon. She had sagging lower eyelids due to excess skin removal from the front of the lower eyelids, scarring behind the eyelids, and weak muscle support. She complained of her cosmetic appearance, and she had irritated eyes from dryness and exposure. In the after photo, she had skin grafting to the back and front of the eyelids and reconstruction of the tendons supporting the eyelids. She is happy with her appearance; and, with proper eyelid placement and function, her eyes are more comfortable.

Facial aging procedures are defined by an approach which
combines restoration of the skin and support to provide
a framework combined with the replacement of lost volume.

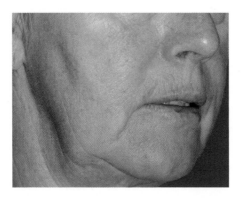

As we get older, the skin, fat and support becomes loose and
stretches, resulting in jowls and loss of definition of the jawline.

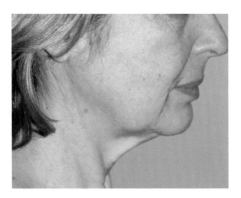

Loosening of neck muscle (called the platysma) and skin result
in the loss of a defined neck angle, occasionally referred to
as a "wattle". Many of our patients schedule consultations
after seeing themselves in a photo or in a dressing room with
a three-way mirror because the wattle appears much larger
from the sides.

Neck Liposculpture

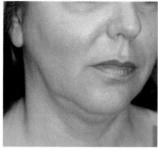
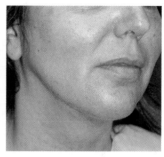

Before   After

For many of our clients, who are in their 30's and 40's, strategic contouring of the neck and jawline with liposuction or laser-assisted liposuction creates a rejuvenated appearance to the neck.

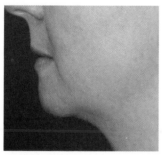
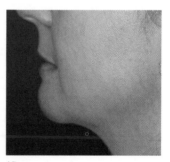

Before   After

A chin implant can permanently balance the profile naturally. Small chins are often associated with "weakness" and "lack of confidence" and can take away from the balance of the face. Chin implants must be reviewed in detail to find the aesthetically most-pleasing size and shape. Selection of the implants is a very involved process and requires a skilled and experienced aesthetic eye.

QUICK RECOVERY FACELIFT

After studying the traditional facelifts' drawbacks, I developed the "Quick Recovery" Facelift. It restores a youthful jawline and allows return to normal activities within a 2-week period. These after views were taken 4 days after the procedure.

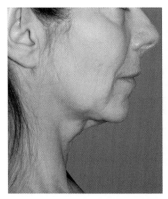
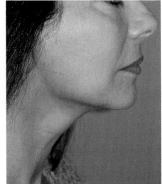

Before

After

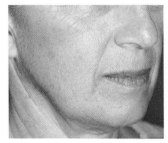
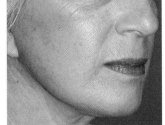

Before

After

THE AGING FACE

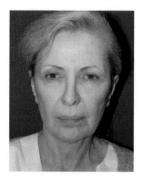

As we age, the face loses the heart shape of youth and becomes more square. As the cheeks become more hollow, jowls form and the neck skin loosens. This results in a change in expression that communicates sadness or lack of energy.

QUICK RECOVERY FACELIFT

Over the past several years, the term "facelift" has been used along with many procedures including creams, injectables, threads, and "miracle" factory procedures sold on infomercials. The modern world's pace leaves little time for long recovery periods. In my practice, I developed "Quick Recovery" techniques and protocols that provide the long-term benefit of traditional procedures with less downtime. This is quite different from most shortcut procedures, which provide little benefit when compared to a properly performed procedure.

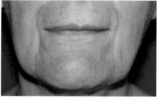 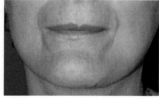

Before   After

This 63 year-old woman had sagging skin and jowls that caused a square shape of the jaw. After facelift surgery, the jawline is a more natural curved shape.

143

RESTORING BALANCE

Approaching facial rejuvenation with the philosophy of doing the least to get the most helps our clients live their busy lives with minimal interruption.

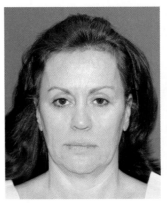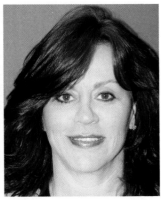

Before   After

A Quick Recovery Face and Neck lift helps change an aged and tired look to an energetic and more youthful appearance.

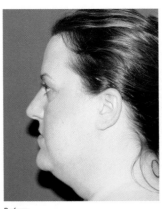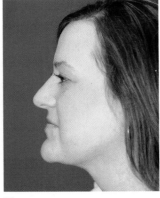

Before   After

CoolLipo™ laser assisted liposculpture helped create a balance between this young woman's face and neck.

144

QUICK RECOVERY LASER PROCEDURES

The Fractional CO2 laser has been a successful technology to help our clients who have sun damaged skin and fine lines as well as deeper wrinkles restore their skin to a more youthful appearance in as little as several days after the procedure.

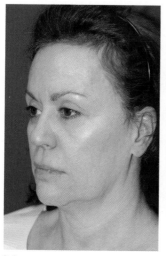 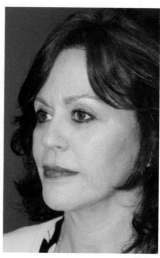

Before   After

Combining Micro Fractional CO2 laser with a Quick Recovery Facelift restored a more youthful face, neck and jawline with smoother and more even toned skin. She was back to work as a Medical Aesthetician within one week.

Neck Bands

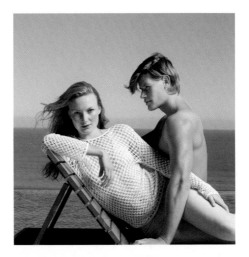

Male models and actors are judged by strong jawlines. The art of restoring facial balance in men is to create a look which is natural and where the incisions are well camouflaged.

QUICK RECOVERY FACELIFT FOR A MALE

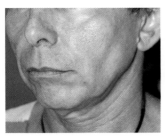

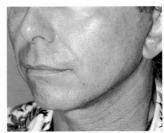

Before   After

This busy professional took very good care of himself but felt that the loose skin at his jawline and neck made him look older. We performed a "small incision" face and neck lift, which resulted in a stronger jawline.

FACELIFT COMPLICATIONS

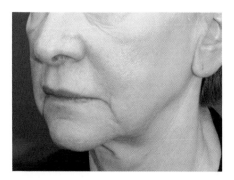

This woman had a "factory" facelift done elsewhere. Within one year of her surgery, her skin sagged and she was disappointed with the result. High volume and high pressure practices frequently perform "1 hour" miracle procedures inappropriately to people who require more time and attention.

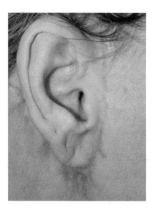

This woman had her facelift surgery by a board certified plastic surgeon whose practice was a high volume/low fee practice. Surgery performed in a rush without proper technique resulted in unsightly scars around her ears that could not be covered with makeup. When she wore earrings, she would draw more attention to this area, making her unable to enjoy her jewelry.

THE HANDS

The hands are often overlooked when people
think about rejuvenating the face. Many of my patients
have commented on how they knew a celebrity
had facial cosmetic surgery because the celebrity's face
looked young but the hands looked "old".
Hand rejuvenation includes procedures such as lasers,
peels, Intense pulsed light (IPL) as well as fillers
such as your own fat. For many of our clients,
it completes the whole picture.

— *Amiya Prasad, M.D., F.A.C.S.*

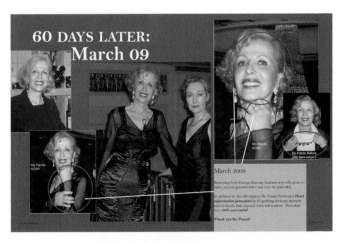

Our patient created a diary of her facial rejuvenation journey
and shows how rejuvenated her hands looked to match her rejuvenated face.

Color versions of the black & white illustrations
found throughout this book
can be found on the following pages

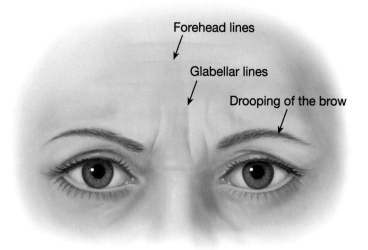

Forehead lines

Glabellar lines

Drooping of the brow

Figure 5-1, page 103

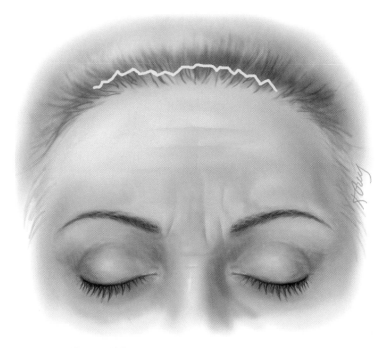

Figure 5-2, page 117

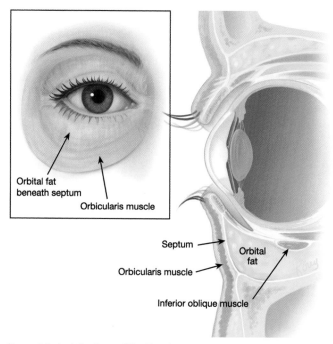

Orbital fat
beneath septum

Orbicularis muscle

Septum

Orbital
fat

Orbicularis muscle

Inferior oblique muscle

Figure 6-1: Architecture of the Eye Area, page 129

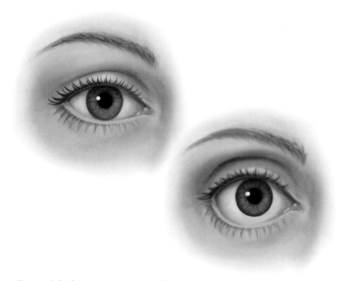

Figure 6-2: Correct iris ratio (left).
Over corrected lid, poor iris ratio (right), page 130

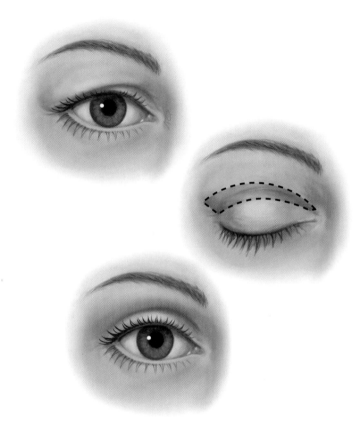

Figure 6-3: Upper lid incision — Before and After, page 136

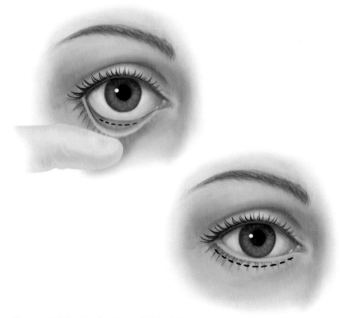

Figure 6-4: Inside-the-lower lid incision, page 140

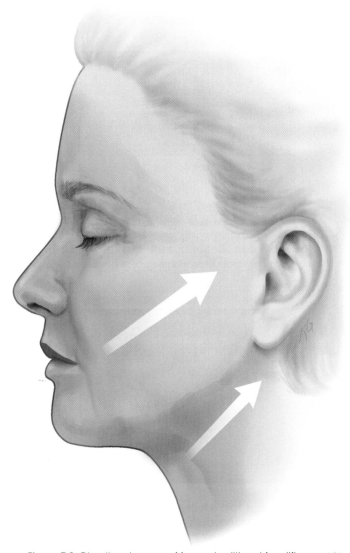

Figure 7-1: Directional arrows of former traditional facelift, page 158

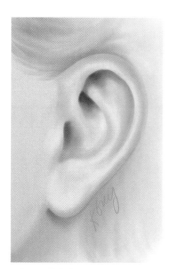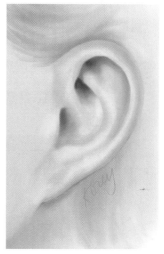

Figure 7-2a, page 161

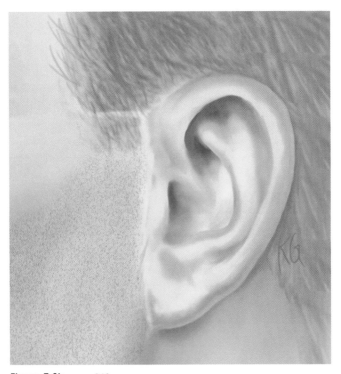

Figure 7-2b, page 163

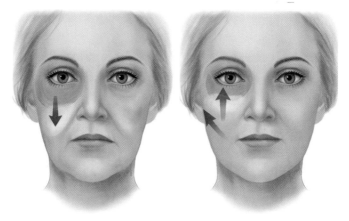

Figure 7-4: Two directions to the mid face lift, page 169

The Fine Art of Looking Younger

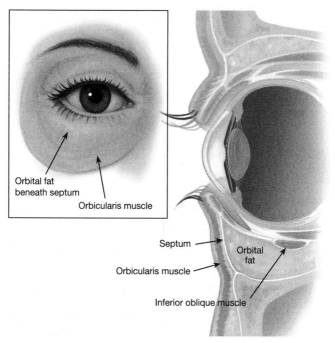

Orbital fat
beneath septum

Orbicularis muscle

Septum

Orbital fat

Orbicularis muscle

Inferior oblique muscle

Figure 6-1: Architecture of the Eye Area

during the removal of lower-eyelid fat. A capable and highly skilled surgeon will avoid compromising the integrity of the muscle to avoid double vision. Lower-eyelid surgery is quite complex, and a great deal of finesse is required in order to maintain the right support to the area and not change the shape of the eye. Normally, the edge of the lower lid is level with the lower margin of the iris, the colored part of the eye. If the support of the lateral lower corner of the eyelid is not maintained, or if too much skin is removed, the desired aesthetic goal is lost. Possibly the patient may require revision surgery to make sure that the eyes don't look old or unnaturally altered after the procedure. Finally, one key aesthetic consideration to eyelid surgery is appreciating how the iris rests in relationship to each eyelid and the white of the eyeball.

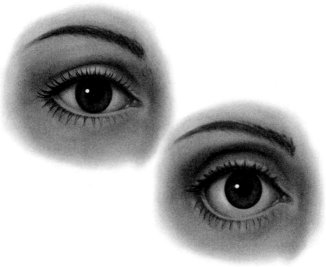

Figure 6-2: Correct iris ratio (left).
Over corrected lid, poor iris ratio (right)

When too much of the white part of the eye, known as the sclera, is visible a condition known as *scleral show* has occurred. Ideally, this condition is avoided through good surgical technique. Scleral show is more common in the traditional external lower lid blepharoplasty and we have performed revision surgery for patients who have come to us under this condition. However, scleral show can occur even when good surgical technique was practiced and the procedure performed was an internal (transconjunctival) lower lid blepharoplasty. The reason is that one cannot always predict patient healing all the time. Scleral show is correctible when it occurs.

Apart from removing fat and repairing muscle, blepharoplasty improves baggy skin under the eyes and corrects sinking upper eyelids or drooping eyelashes that impair vision. The surgery can sometimes treat a medical condition called ptosis — drooping eyelid — which is caused by weak muscle tone or nerve damage. However in many cases, ptosis repair calls for repair of the eyelid muscle itself. This fact may be lost on the general plastic surgeon, although it is one of the procedures that oculofacial plastic surgeons concentrate on. Many times people are told that a blepharoplasty will fix the drooping problem only to discover after surgery that the ptosis recurs because the muscle was not repaired. Ptosis causes the eyelids to hang very low, which can block vision. The condition results when the "lifting" muscle (known as the levator muscle) simply stretches and thins. Many sufferers are frustrated by the strain of keeping their eyes open, particularly when reading. They will complain of headaches, because they inadvertently raise their eyebrows to get some lift on their lids. This action contributes to a tension headache when the forehead muscles are raised for long periods. Changing eyeglasses and cataract surgery can't possibly resolve the problem. Often patients wrongly presume that their eyes have gotten smaller. Fortunately, ptosis repair allows patients to see better and to look better, and many times successful surgery will improve the character of the face. As a reminder: *Blepharoplasty does not treat drooping eyebrows or facial and brow wrinkles. These are best addressed by facelift and browlift surgeries that can ameliorate this type of facial sagging.* Also, eyelid surgery will not correct dark circles. Dark circles can be treated with other approaches, such as creams containing hydroquinone or azeleic acid and a well-designed skin-care regimen that involves adequate moisturizing. If you are fair-skinned, certain laser treatments may be an option for you. One caution: laser treatments to treat dark circles on patients with dark skin could worsen the situation. How then to best rejuvenate your eyes? Let's begin with nonsurgical options and then explore upper and lower eyelifts.

Wan and Hollowed Eyes

Youthful eyes feature a certain dewy suppleness that is created by a general distribution of healthy volume throughout the area. When this volume — mostly fat — is depleted in the upper area, eyes take on a wan look. At times the eye socket and bony understructure are more apparent. The absence of volume in the lower region results in a hollowed look. While puffy eyes suggest tiredness, hollowed eyes impart a sickly demeanor. The wan appearance may be further exaggerated by other anatomical factors, such as poor bony formation below the eye or the downward drift of the fat and muscles of the cheek. Overzealous cosmetic surgery is another culprit. A hollowed expression occurs when too much of the orbital fat is removed. Genetic traits play a role, especially among young patients. How then to restore a more youthful, supple contour? Dermal fillers, injected beneath the skin via a fine needle, help replace soft tissue volume loss. These fillers come in a wide range of consistencies across a myriad of brand names. Another choice is to undergo a "fat transfer.," This utilizes the patient's own fat , which has been specially treated. Fat transfers deliver better results where the skin is thicker, such as the cheek; they're not optimal for thin-skinned areas under the eyes. Also, fat transfers often are slightly less predictable, and many patients require more than one treatment. *It is crucial to understand that precision and protection of the eye are vital.* You need a highly skilled surgeon to deliver seamless and beautiful results. In some cases, "sculpting" the area with fillers is required, so an aesthetic sensibility coupled with expertise deliver optimum results. Fillers can be used in the lower eyelid, cheek junction, and tear trough to transform the area. Patients across all age groups have enjoyed beautiful results via volume augmentation. The major drawback to fillers is their impermanence. Each patient has a varying response. Some may last for almost a year and some as little as six months. It is a personal choice and one best made with the advice of an expert surgeon.

Deep Wrinkles

Sometimes when people smile, they develop a fold right underneath the lashes of the lower eyelid. This is a contraction of the *orbicularis oculi* muscle, which goes around the orbit of the eye. The muscle is thickened over time and can be readily corrected with a tiny amount of Botox. By paralyzing just a few fibers of this muscle, one loses the thickness and hypertrophy seen when smiling. Crow's-feet caused by muscle movement will be inhibited by Botox, making the area appear relaxed. Following Botox, supplemental laser therapy can smooth area lines. In combination, this nonsurgical twosome imparts a rejuvenated glow to the face.

Fine Wrinkles

Fine lines tend to form under the eyelids, and most are typical of static wrinkles that develop from aging and sun exposure. Smoking, excessive eye rubbing, and stress also contribute to fine lines as well as to dark circles. Because the lines are delicate, lasers and chemical peels often deliver the best results. Today's innovative lasers, particularly the state-of-the-art microfractional CO_2 laser, which I prefer, allow clients to heal faster than ever. This laser is considerably gentler to the skin than other resurfacing lasers. It stimulates the production of collagen, which results in a tightening and smoothing of the skin. Most people are able to return to their normal activities in about one week after this type of laser skin treatment. During this period, topical ointments are applied to allow the skin to heal as soon as possible — but the unpleasant angry red patches and longer periods of healing associated with earlier lasers are gone. Makeup can usually be worn one week later. The overall appearance continues to improve with time. Additionally, aesthetic techniques can be adapted by a skilled surgeon who knows how to manipulate lasers effectively. This artistic adaptation dramatically improves the texture and smoothness of the skin.

Upper Eyelid Blepharoplasty

For many patients, excess skin on the upper eyelids is frustrating. Runners find the skin can be irritated by sweat. Eye rubbing only exacerbates the itchiness. Female patients discover that applying makeup becomes problematic. The goal of upper-lid surgery is to restore the lid's natural line and

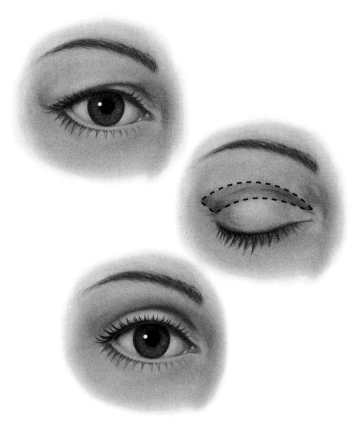

Figure 6-3: Upper lid incision — Before and After

impart a rested, refreshed appearance. Generally, this is done via excising the precisely correct amount of loose, extra skin. If too much skin is removed, some patients are unable to close their eyes and the expression at rest is unnatural.

I have developed techniques in blepharoplasty surgery that involve minimal incisions and local anesthesia to deliver a very natural result. My approach differs from traditional eyelid blepharoplasty surgery. First, it involves minimal risk, uses minimal anesthesia, and — this is the best part — the outcome offers truly maximal aesthetic results. Through the minimal incision, excess fat and tissue is removed, the skin and muscle are re-draped, and the incision is sutured closed. There tends to be less bruising with this technique.

Local anesthesia with sedation as needed means less downtime after the procedure, a clear advantage over general anesthesia. The latter has more attendant risks, and there is a higher incidence of nausea. Thus, generally speaking, local anesthesia offers a safer option. The scar heals extremely well and is virtually imperceptible even when the eyes are closed.

Lower-Eyelid Blepharoplasty

Lower-eyelid blepharoplasty is performed to modify puffy bags, loose skin, and sagging tissue supporting the lower eyelids. Under-eye puffiness typically stems from fatty deposits beneath the skin. The eye sits in a space called the orbit, and when we're young, the resilient orbital septum holds the fat deposits in place. These fat deposits are necessary to cushion the eyeball in the orbit. However, over time the orbital septum, a fibrous membrane wall, loses some of its structural integrity. As it weakens, fat pushes forward — bulging, in a sense. Puffy bags result. Unfortunately, this type of bulging can be inherited and may start as early as adolescence.

Additionally, the fatty tissue holds water. That's why, in the morning, after you've reclined all night, eyelids may appear at their puffiest. Over the course of the day, gravity (and circulation) will help drain some of the fluid. Still, like delicate eye tissue that becomes increasingly lax through the years, puffiness eventually prevails. The added fluid pressure over time exacerbates the delicate structure, which adds to an aged appearance.

By understanding how the underlying structure changes through the years, you can see why a weak membrane *inside of the eyelid* will never be healed by a topical eye cream, no matter how costly. Creams may make the skin *appear* smoother. But the underlying source of puffiness needs to be treated via surgery.

There are several different surgical techniques that a physician can use to rejuvenate lower lids. The overall approach usually involves removing fat (or sculpting and redistributing the fat or septum) as well as removing excess skin and muscle. Two of the more popular approaches are described below.

Lower-Lid Incision

The majority of practitioners use an external incision, just below the eyelashes. Known as the *transcutaneous* incision — meaning through the skin — this provides access to the underlying tissue so that fat can be manipulated and excess skin can be tightened. If the incision is well placed, no visible scar is evident after healing. However, patients with darker skin may experience darker pigmentation along the incision line. This approach may also be associated with scleral show, where too much of the eye's white area is evident. Possibly the lower eyelid may turn outward, resulting in an unattractive *ectropion* condition, which can exacerbate dry eyes. The surgery demands precise and careful manipulation of the delicate muscle that serves as a supporting "hammock." This is a fragile area, and if the integrity is compromised, the shape of the eye can be unfortunately altered. This method is a good approach for people with fragile skin that is thin and papery. Although I prefer the technique described below, there are people who would do better with a transcutaneous approach. I advise people with Northern European skin, who have more of a tendency to develop thin skin as they age, to seek out rejuvenation procedures earlier rather than later. In this way, they can benefit from the transconjunctival method described next.

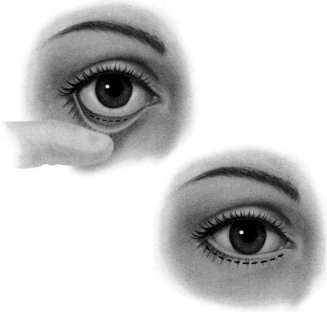

Figure 6-4: Inside-the-lower lid incision

Inside-the-Lid Incision

I prefer to use an internal incision known as the *transconjunctival* incision — meaning *inside* the eyelid. This incision offers clear benefits: There are no outside scars, and the shape of the eye is typically better preserved. It also reduces trauma to the fragile support network that must maintain the integrity of the eye. There is a great deal of discussion in the cosmetic surgery medical literature as to how to attach the point of the lateral *canthus* (the outer corner of the eye). This is a crucial step and is done once the lower lid has been adjusted with the right amount of fat manipulation. The goal of the cosmetic repair is to maximally rejuvenate the eye with long-lasting results. Many surgeons write about specific techniques, but in reality, each patient has an individual curve and eye shape.

No single technique can consistently offer the best results. I have found that true artistry comes from mastering the various surgical options and then deciding how to execute a particular technique so that the balance of the face is preserved. In this way, the rejuvenated face appears natural. If you were to ask a portrait painter how colors are chosen for skin tones, an amateur might claim peach tones work best for a light-skinned person and brown tones better match a darker complexion. But this is an absurd oversimplification. True artists work with a myriad of pigments, blending a wide variety on a palette that is highly individualized, unique to each artist. Only a skilled portrait painter can effectively capture the brilliancy, transparency and wide variables that reflect the subject's skin tone. The same can be said of a skilled surgeon; each identifies which technique will best rejuvenate a patient's eyes.

Because the eyelid is not "taken apart" from the outside or front, it is easier for me to gauge the effect of fat removal as the operation is in progress. This permits me to have a more accurate assessment of the amount of fat to be sculpted. I view this as a superior surgery, depending on the right candidate, because its nature permits more precision. Since the operation does not cut the delicate middle layer of the eyelid, the possibility of scar contractions that alter the shape do not develop. This contraction might occur immediately after surgery but also may present itself years later. Since the approach is less invasive, there is generally less bruising and swelling.

Misguided surgeons can excise too much fat, which traumatizes the area, and the eyes do not look refreshed once recovery has occurred. In addition to perfecting minimally invasive techniques, with the benefits of less healing time and more natural results, I have developed a highly individualized screening system for blepharoplasty prospects. One may properly classify a person's unique features and eyelids on the basis of gender, age, ethnic background and skin condition. This analysis is unique, another point of difference I offer, and it allows me to select the right approach that is properly personalized to your unique needs. It is a useful tool, but the personalized artistic touch I bring to your special situation is what makes all the difference in the beauty of your results. This aesthetic interpretation is often overlooked by other surgeons, and I urge you to seek those surgeons who are guided by a refined aesthetic ability.

General Length of Surgery

Average eyelid surgery may last one to two hours, depending on the extent of treatment. Prior to the start of your procedure, the treatment area will be cleansed and anesthesia will be administered. In general, local anesthesia can be used with sedation, in which the eyelids and surrounding areas are numb and you are in a relaxed state. General anesthesia, in which you are asleep, can induce nausea during the immediate recovery, and it seems an excessive step for most patients. General anesthesia often represents a greater convenience for the surgeon, but it may represent a greater burden to the patient.

Bruising and swelling are likely after surgery and tend to diminish within a week to ten days. Stitches, usually of the absorbable type, typically dissolve by one week. Thereafter, patients may wear makeup. Also, a good pair of sunglasses will go a long way. In our office, we offer state-of-the-art mineral-based makeup that makes a tremendous difference in the cover-up. Contact lenses can usually be worn in about two weeks. Most people return to work in about a week. Finally, with both upper-lid and lower-lid surgery, a few medical conditions make blepharoplasty more risky. These include thyroid problems such as hypothyroidism and Graves' disease, dry eye or lack of sufficient tears, high blood pressure or other circulatory disorders, cardiovascular disease, and diabetes. If you have an eye-related condition, such as Graves' disease or dry eye, my expertise as an oculofacial plastic surgeon allows me to advise you and discuss alternative treatments and surgical procedures, if necessary. A patient must have sufficient structure to support the procedure. It's important to be completely honest about all medications and herbal supplements; these can impede surgery and compromise your healing period.

Chapter Six

Male Eyes Have Unique Challenges

Only an experienced specialist knows how to differentiate the techniques used in male blepharoplasty from those used on female eyes. It is a crucial and absolutely necessary distinction. For a man's rejuvenation procedure to succeed, the patient must retain his masculine expression. Additionally, the integrity of his masculine look must be preserved via individual facial characteristics and attributes that are also sex specific. A generic and stereotypical feminine eye contour simply reduces a man to a softer caricature of himself. Usually the candidate doesn't look refreshed. Instead, he looks somewhat transgendered. For instance, a man's upper-eyelid crease is lower than that of a woman. Also, the line of a male eyebrow is somewhat straighter, more level. If these contours are not preserved during blepharoplasty, a man not only loses his individuality but assumes a more feminine expression.

Many surgeons mistakenly over correct the male eyelid, eradicating those subtle distinctions that are handsome and convey a certain ruggedness. A quick search of male celebrities in the media — especially male rock and pop stars — easily illustrates how generic rejuvenation, when performed by the wrong surgeon, erases masculinity.

Some of these surgeons were no doubt sought out for their fine reputations. But their "red carpet" publicity likely stemmed from successful cosmetic surgery on younger female pop stars or older actresses. To me, their work misses the masculine mark. Also, when a patient lives in the limelight, misguided surgeons erroneously seek to remove *all* signs of aging. Over-correction often creates an artificially round eye, much like that of a doll. That's when the unfortunate headlines follow, geared to sell magazine copies with cover blurbs that announce Botched Plastic Surgery or Celebrity Surgery Disasters.

I strongly urge all male candidates to find a surgeon with deep experience in rejuvenating men's eyes. Study the Before and After images. See if you can view a successful result where the patient's features are similar to yours and the final results matches your goals. Remember that male eyes need to have a relaxed, masculine quality in order to maintain a natural appearance. Find a surgeon who can capably differentiate what sex specific variables must be considered and how specific approaches can be adapted for your male aesthetic needs.

Ethnic Eye Procedures

The Asian eyelid is different in many ways, which is why specialized eyelid surgery is necessary to yield natural results. One of the more inappropriate aesthetic applications used by misguided plastic surgeons in the past was "Americanizing" or "Europeanizing" the beautiful Asian eyelid. Asian eyes require delicate finesse in treating the typical *epicanthal* fold that lies in front of the eye. In this way, a natural and appropriate rejuvenation will be enhanced in line with the standards of Asian beauty. Asian individuals may also benefit from the "double eyelid fold" procedure. This protects the inherent attractiveness of the Asian eye while giving the upper eyelid a visible crease when the eye is open. This change to the upper eyelid makes it easier to apply makeup and is considered to be a desirable aesthetic appearance in many Asian cultures.

Because skin comes in a variety of shades, dark-skinned people should be aware that certain incisions heal differently. Blepharoplasty has a variety of important ethnic considerations, and skin color is one. Dark skin has more melanin (with the added benefit of greater sun protection and less wrinkling!), but facial incisions can thicken. An incision that is not skillfully executed may result in a more visible scar. And generally, incisions on darker skin are slightly thicker than those found on lighter, paler complexions. When a scar continues to grow

179

during and beyond the healing period, keloids may develop. These are scars that are thick and large, and they can continue to enlarge if left untreated. Fortunately, keloids are very rare in properly performed ethnic eye cosmetic surgery.

I prefer to deploy very fine instruments, lasers, and radio frequency wave procedures, all of which minimize the risk of keloids after surgery. In addition, good clinical judgment dictates conservative skin removal, low tension on the scars, and sub-cuticular repair in the dermis with minimal skin stitches. These will reduce the chance of keloid formation even further.

Are You A Candidate?

There are a few signs to help guide you toward or away from eye rejuvenation. I find these questions help address your concerns.

◆ Do people always ask if you're tired, even when you get plenty of sleep?

◆ Do the bags under your eyes, which used to vanish by the morning shower, now stay throughout the day?

◆ Do you work in an image-driven industry, one where you may need to project a lot of energy?

- Is applying makeup increasingly difficult?

- Do foundation and eye shadow tend to crease following application and when you smile?

- Are you buying different creams and gels to improve the way your eyes look, but find they're ineffective?

- Are you self-conscious when readying to embark on a new phase or job?

- Would looking more refreshed help you feel more confident?

- Do you exercise and eat right, but your eyes don't look as good as you feel?

- Do you worry about feeling less attractive when you look in the mirror?

- Are you surprised by the appearance of your eyes when you look at photographs of yourself?

If you find you've answered "yes" to several questions, why not discuss possible options with a qualified surgeon? During your consultation, be sure to determine if your surgeon is compassionate, caring, and genuinely concerned about your needs. Your surgeon should be your trustworthy guide on the path to reach your aesthetic goals.

Quick Review

◆ Today's best cosmetic blepharoplasty procedures are built around a modern understanding of eyelid and facial aging. Choose only a skilled surgeon who uses state-of-the-art surgeries, one who understands the eyelids' complex system of support and the perils of disturbing orbital fat .

◆ Do your research. Understand what you may realistically expect from each procedure.

◆ Puffy lids — upper and lower — can now be addressed surgically with less tissue disruption and scarring, thereby yielding both a more pleasing enhancement and a safer long-term result.

◆ Since the eyes truly individualize your appearance, *it's crucial to carefully select the most qualified surgeon you can find.* One of the more common complaints among dissatisfied blepharoplasty patients is, "I don't look like myself anymore." If finding a skilled surgeon means traveling to another city, state, or country, then travel!

◆ Understand the crucial importance of skilled experience when selecting your surgeon. Even a nearly imperceptible "slightly misguided incision" may leave the eyes and lids looking harsh, surprised, hollowed, and wan. 🦎

"Beautiful young people are accidents of nature, but beautiful old people are works of art"

— Eleanor Roosevelt
First Lady of the United States,
1933-1943

CHAPTER SEVEN

A Better Facelift

Nearly any evening news program offers late breaking stories about the most recent pharmaceutical advancements or innovative scientific discoveries. Cosmetic surgery has its share of newsworthy breakthroughs, though it also has its fair share of hype — without heft. About every six months there's some consumer buzz on a new, "never before heard from," "cutting edge," "state of the art," "technological breakthrough" way to get full facelift results *with no surgery.* Witness the popularity of such cosmetics as "eyelifts in a bottle," "facelift in a bottle," "liquid facelift," and my personal favorite, "plastic surgeon in a bottle." When patients with significant facial aging ask about a minilift, I have to tell them, "A mini facelift means mini results."

From my earliest days as a fellow, I was driven by a belief that the traditional facelift could deliver superior results. However, there were aspects that I felt needed to change. How best to reduce the bruising? What would shorten the average recovery time? The traditional facelift prevailed during those days but these disturbing issues continued to prey upon my mind. For the most part, the traditional facelift is still used by "big name" surgeons whose schedules are driven by four or six month wait lists. The dilemma continues: When a surgeon is completely booked, and the future is filled with appointments, is he or she able to take time off to study or perfect newer and superior techniques? Not really. No surprise then, that many practices throughout the US and Europe eventually evolve into assembly line productions.

Lesser known surgeons readily use the traditional approach as well, since they assume it represents the "choice" of many surgeons it must be the best approach, right? Unfortunately, no. This one-size-fits-all facelift surgery is the reason why more patients end up with unnatural results. We can all easily picture these unfortunate results among well known celebrities. They are not exempt. In fact, they are often the targets of the paparazzi, precisely because they had bad plastic surgery. Popular weekly magazines appear to gloat over "botched" movie star cosmetic surgeries gone wrong. There are websites devoted just to this aspect of popular culture and many are heavily trafficked. We all know the axiom: 'If it's not broke, don't fix it.' Truth? Facelifts needed a fix for a long time.

What Needed To Change?

Over the years, the majority of cosmetic surgeons appeared to agree that gravity caused a general downward collapse of youthful contours. There's truth to this premise, though some research suggests gravity alone does not create this downward shift. That's because we are learning how the face, made up of individual fat compartments, loses and gains fat at different rates. So both volume loss and gravity actually create the aging dynamic. Nevertheless, it was the goal of the traditional facelift to defy this downward progression by attempting to "lift" the fallen tissues. In simplest terms, a traditional facelift sought to eliminate sagging and wrinkles. The arrows in the illustration below (Figure 7-1) show how in the traditional face lift facial tissue was lifted *outward* to the ears.

Through the years, advances permitted surgeons to reach deeper into the underlying facial tissue structure. Yet, even in the hands of a skilled surgeon, the deeper and more extensive the reach of a facelift, the greater the risks. More bruising resulted and greater recovery time was necessary. Fat, often viewed to be an aging culprit, was also removed, making eyes appear hollowed and sunken. Over time, as eliminating wrinkles became the "gold standard," an exaggerated, distorted result evolved. Increasingly there were more instances of an unfortunate and unnatural "pulled look." My personal philosophy *is that no one should notice cosmetic surgery; no one should compliment your facelift.* Results should be natural and youthful. A patient should emerge, after full recovery,

appearing natural and feeling more youthful. All worthy goals.
All natural results. It's what several of my patients have called

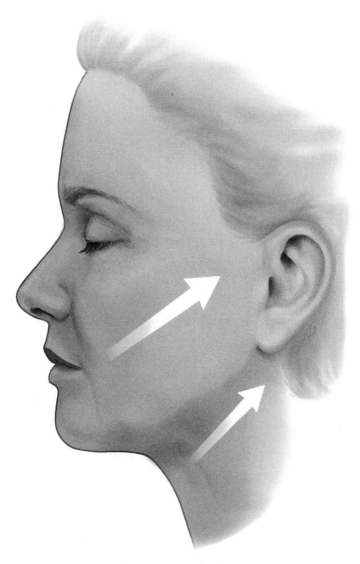

Figure 7-1: Directional arrows of former traditional facelift.

"the Prasad point of difference." As you explore cosmetic surgery, stay focused on finding the best qualified surgeon to create a natural looking appearance *for you.* Each surgery must be individualized.

When I am asked to do corrective work, it's not unusual for a concerned family member to accompany the new patient. This can be a tough part of any initial consultation. Their dismay and angst is as palpable as that of the prospective patient. A question often begins the consultation, "Will she look like herself again?" And I know exactly what they mean without even studying the Before photos. The concerned family member is uneasy with the appearance of afraid or uneven eyes, or a perpetually surprised expression, even a too wide 'frog' mouth. Often there is a pulled and tight expression that may persist. While these unfortunate results may occur for a variety of misguided reasons, often they are attributed to the surgeon's personal drive to eliminate all wrinkles, at practically any cost. These unfortunate results also suggest that the surgeon simply does not appreciate or understand the role of deflation, or facial volume loss, which this chapter helps explain.

The Earlobe Dilemma

Before we move to the challenge of how to successfully ameliorate deflation, there is yet another undesirable and unnatural facelift outcome you need to know about. In this area, you'll need to develop a very keen eye so you can protect yourself against ear lobe complications. Surprisingly, it is not consistently addressed in consultations and there doesn't seem to be much medical coverage about the high percentage of unsatisfactory results in this crucial area. Thus, it's up to you to screen your surgeon candidate carefully for a successful outcome.

When surgery requires an outward "lift," often the original position of ears must be modified and thus the final placement may be compromised. In many cases it is the ear's appearance *after a facelift* that may betray a natural appearance. An unnatural outcome may develop when there's a downward pull of the earlobe; the final appearance is at odds with a younger face. However, apart from the ear's unnatural appearance, often it's how the ear *feels* to the patient that can create major discomfort.

One of the more common complaints with new patients seeking corrective work is that their ears feel awkward. It's not that these patients feel pain. They don't. But an unnatural and distracting feeling plagues them daily. After a lifetime of never thinking about their ears, now they are unable to wear highly prized earrings. Or a phone no longer rests comfortably for easy listening. If you think this is a superficial concern, place a small piece of tape around a portion of your ear and try to muscle through the day. Since ears vary widely, your surgeon will require a superior skill set to make sure he preserves the features you have. In some aging individuals, the earlobes may elongate.

Few facelift surgeries will attempt to modify the ear's proportion although it takes a skilled surgeon little time to reduce the

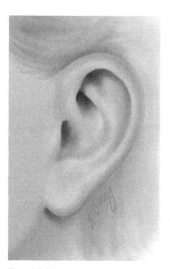 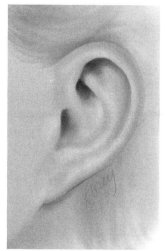

Figure 7-2a

earlobe size. This step makes the ear as rejuvenated as the face. It is something you should ask about because it may be important, even crucial, to the overall successful outcome of your facelift. With other patients, lobes become creased with aging, often an inherited trait. Thus, while the face appears rejuvenated, ears may belie a more youthful appearance. Other earlobe challenges can arise when there's an excessive skin excision around the earlobe during a face-lift. Men have special earlobe aesthetic needs in order to successfully accommodate a facelift. In an earlier section, I describe the trichophytic incision for browlifts. This same incision is equally superior for lifts to the midface region in the right candidate.

It is surprising that many patients who come to me for revision surgery have no clue as to where the original incision was to made. They never asked! In the two sketches below (Figure 7-2a and 7-2b), you can see how distortions easily may result. I urge you to carefully study the earlobe results of any surgeon's Before and After photos *before you make a choice*. Screen your surgeon about your ear concerns. Please don't accept a pat, "Don't worry, it will be fine." Ask. Most patients tend to pore over eyes, chin and smile features in Before and After photos. They'll study the wrinkles. *Study earlobe placement as well.*

Earlobes, like noses, have a wide range of shapes and sizes. So the skilled surgeon must consider each individual's earlobe idiosyncrasies. In this way, the best final result will leave the lobe in a natural position, one that matches the patient's more youthful and refreshed appearance.

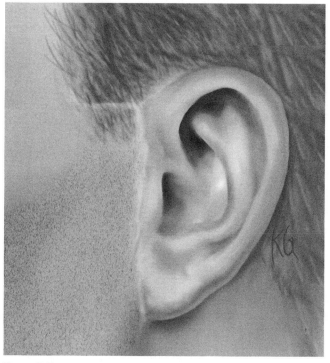

Figure 7-2b

A More Natural Lift:
What the Old Masters Taught Me

During my training, colleagues and I would attend the patients of seasoned surgeons, following procedures. We'd look for hematomas, make sure no patient had 'popped' their stitches. We'd remove drains and — if all went well — we'd re-wrap the patient with fresh mummy-like bandages. I'd even sketch possible approaches to make a less invasive incision, wondering if there were a way to "do less," but deliver "more."

Once I had my own practice, the well being and aesthetic goals of my patients were paramount. Training as an oculofacial surgeon had its advantages. One benefit is that I was able to minimize post surgery bruising very early on. Busy executives helped build my practice through word of mouth. Technical instruments improved over time and significant quantum leaps could be made with lasers.

Any new "surgical option" creates a flurry of consumer interest and most, such as the thread lift, gave me pause. The thread lift is a quick outpatient procedure in which doctors "thread" serrated plastic sutures through the fatty layer beneath the face and use them to hoist sagging tissue. The idea is to pull the skin taut, so the face looks smoother and more youthful. The thread lift sounds interesting but one has to ask, "What if a patient were especially expressive or animated, won't the threads feel strange? Might they dislodge?" Yes, to both questions. Thus the benefit of the procedure are lost. Not surprisingly, thread lifts have fallen out of favor and are hardly ever performed anymore. And as helpful as Botox or Dysport can be, there's only so much of a surgeon can use to control expressions before the patient's face becomes an inanimate stone mask.

Surgeons often are compelled to pore over medical journals. Frequently, the articles are illustrated with a variety of medical photographs or highly detailed illustrations. These updates are invaluable but there are limits to what an illustration can accurately portray. So, to my surprise, it was an artist who lived centuries ago who also taught me a great lesson. I still love to sketch faces and I enjoy studying portrait painting by exceptional artists such as Rembrandt and Velázquez. These Old Masters painted multiple portraits of a single person over a lifetime. In those days, there were no cameras to capture the person's likeness. So while it is likely there was a stand-in for a King or Pope when the artist painted the lace collar, there was no substitute for the aging face of Spain's King Philip IV. He had to show up. And Velázquez had to paint him.

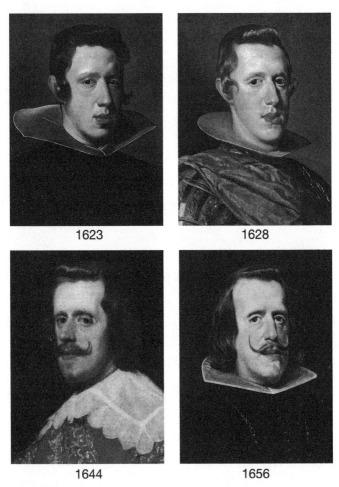

1623   1628

1644   1656

Figure 7-3

It is through Velásquez's genius and clever use of rich pigments that I made a discovery. This court painter's brush strokes communicated a subtle understanding of "facial deflation" through the years. His work reveals more to me about facial aging than many modern photographs or medical illustrations possibly could. His skill as a court painter proves that what typifies an older face is the loss of youthful plumpness. *Aging is less about lines and wrinkles and more about general deflation or overall facial volume loss.* It's as simple as that. For decades, cosmetic facial surgery focused on eradicating wrinkles. It failed to adequately address the loss of facial volume, except for the occasional use of injectable filler where post surgical lines would prevail. But this dual approach — lifting outward and then filling lines — has limits.

Today we know that the cell's ability to hold water within its wall is weakened over time and, as we age, our cells 'spring' microscopic leaks. No longer water logged, cells deflate and by our fifth decade, the average person loses as much as 30% (or more) of water when compared to those of a twenty year old. Bone loss also progresses through the years. *This attrition is revealed by studying the subtle shifts in facial planes through the decades.* While we surgeons use Before and After photos to record patient progress, photography is unable to tell a complete story. Each single image only captures a person's expression *at the very second the shutter is pressed.* A person's face, young or old, is about features and facial planes, and it is the latter that the flash of a camera tends to flatten. This photographic flatness tends to distort reality, too. I think that's why there are some people look better than others when photographed.

While I studied Velásquez's younger portraits of King Philip IV, I had an epiphany. An Old Master oil portrait reveals a truth that a camera cannot capture. An Old Master portrait captures a fuller range of human nuances; it reveals a *fluid expression*. Perhaps this is why the Mona Lisa by daVinci continues to be studied and debated and admired: she's smiling. But what exactly is she thinking? And if you move around this portrait in the Louvre, her eyes seem to follow you. Her expression changes. This just does not happen with medical photographs, even if a world-class photographer snapped the images! And so it was through a study of Old master portraits, and their flow of expressions, that one sees the more subtle nuances of aging due to deflation.

Additionally, the richness of the Old Master painter's pigments, unlike drier palettes of more modern painters (and today's modern digital camera), heighten a depth and translucence that only reveal themselves when one studies the face. This translucence shifts over time. Yet it makes each face unique and truly human. So what did Velázquez teach me? A lot. His portraits revealed the limitations of the traditional approach favored by most surgeons. Lifting outward toward the ears does nothing to ameliorate the loss of volume, no matter how deeply the surgeon may go to excise excess tissue. In fact, in some cases it can make a person's face more narrow and angular. If there was a way to reposition the deflated fat and tissues closer to their more youthful repose, wouldn't the facelift deliver superior results? I was excited that the precision of my oculofacial training could be deployed in a new and innovative manner.

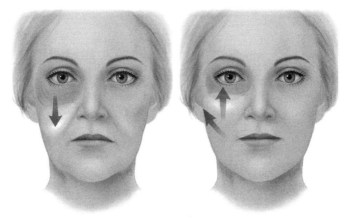

Figure 7-4: Two directions to the mid face lift

A Different Direction

Facial fat, once viewed as an undesirable aging by-product, a commodity that should be removed, now might achieve a better status. It could help restore a certain degree of facial volume by simply re-shifting its position. A side benefit to this new perspective is that by moving these fatty pads upwards to distinct compartments in the cheek area will result in an upward migration that will help eliminate lines around the nose and mouth. And equally important is that this repositioning improves volume loss under the eyes. The results are exciting. By elevating the fallen compartments upward, there is even the potential of adding more curve to the upper lip or reducing the downward curve of the upper lip, which sometimes occurs as we age. This upward shift restores a more youthful appearance to the face.

As this illustration shows, there are two directions to the mid face lift. The first arrow indicates an "outward" direction, like the more traditional lift. The second "upward" arrow indicates a meaningful point of difference. It is this maneuver that gives better rejuvenation by restoring volume.

Nose to Mouth Creases

When patients are dissatisfied with the results from a traditional facelift, often they complain about "those lines," tracing a straight finger from the nose down to the mouth to demonstrate the line that bothers them most. As one patient lamented, "After surgery, the two creases are still there and no amount of cover up makes those lines go away." In cosmetic surgery, those lines are known as "nasolabial folds." And often their presence following facelift surgery disappoints patients. As with all cosmetic procedures, successful remedies depend on several factors. Skin elasticity and thickness may play a role in how deeply these creases appear.

I have found that by lifting the cheek pads with a mid face lift, most patients will enjoy a superior result. By lifting upwards, fullness softens the creases. The upward direction delivers a more youthful, refreshed appearance. In addition, there are non-invasive remedies which can help minimize nasolabial lines such as fillers, even nasolabial implants, typically inserted through an incision inside the mouth. I urge you to seek a variety of opinions over several consultations to help determine your best option.

Cheek Enhancement

I recall reading that we Americans apparently top all other cultures in the consumption of bronzers and cheek blush. Apparently we spend millions of dollars beyond what other countries invest — perhaps we recognize how the appearance of rosy, plump cheeks actually conveys a sense of youth and robust health.

Some patients believe injectable fillers or fat transfers may be used as an effective means to add volume to cheeks. Although I do offer this to patients who elect this choice, I do like to discuss the utility of implants. The key rationale is that injectable supplements do not deliver a long term cheek remedy. A good deal of filler may be required to create fullness and the long term cost is significant when compared to an implant. Cosmetic surgery is about choices, and my experience suggests cheek implants are quite successful across a wide variety of patients; the procedure offers a realistic, and natural result with longer term benefits.

The first question most patients ask about cheek augmentation is: "What's the difference between malar and sub malar implants?" To keep it simple:

♦ The malar region is the outer upper cheek area that imparts a sculpted or 'chiseled' appearance of high cheekbones.

♦ The submalar region is the lower or mid-cheek area. This region often sinks or appears gaunt, frequently from aging, though many younger patients simply lack an average amount of cheek definition. Flatness in the midface region, for younger patients, tends to be hereditary, though long distance joggers and serious athletes may also develop a hollowed look as body fat diminishes.

Since the aesthetic goal of this specific surgery seeks to create greater definition, a successful result can offer an appealing and very natural enhancement. In general, implants vary in size and shape and are made of silicone. Once the correct implant is selected to match the aesthetic goal, the surgery is conducted through incisions made inside the mouth, above the upper gums. I prefer 'twilight' sedation for quick recovery

This is where the skilled surgeon carefully manipulates the implant into the precisely perfect location, being exceedingly careful to enhance the appearance, revealing the ideal of facial symmetry that is nonetheless natural. For the most part, the surgery takes about an hour.

Laser Enhancements With a Facelift

Prior to the microfractional CO_2 laser, it was unsafe to laser the skin during a facelift. But the microfractional CO_2 laser changes this shortcoming by leaving superficial skin intact; there's no additional healing delay to this type of laser treatment. While the facelift repositions loose skin and muscle to restore youthful facial planes, if the skin has fine lines, sun spots, blemishes, deep lines on the cheeks, or acne scars and pits, then laser enhancement will remedy these problems, leaving skin smooth and glowing. The advantage of having both procedures simultaneously is that healing times are also simultaneous. In addition, the CO_2 Laser is quite efficacious; most patients require a single treatment to achieve the results that they seek. I have included this information here because it is very important to understand what a facelift will do for you and what other procedures will make the lift complete, imparting the desired appearance.

The Neck

The neck's muscles also eventually succumb to a loss of firmness. As neck muscles become loose and drop underneath the skin, the flaccid result can make us appear older. In some cases, the mid face lift can ameliorate a patient's neck contour, delivering good results. In other instances, a separate procedure is required to deliver a more youthful appearance. Also, significant fat under the chin, often an inherited trait, can rob a person of a youthful appearance. To eliminate excess chin fat, liposuction can make a remarkable correction. Access is made via a small incision under the chin, virtually imperceptible once healed.

Aside from liposuction, neck tissue that is considerably loose and sagging is best ameliorated by a necklift specific to the person's aesthetic goals. The necklift, if done in tandem with a facelift, can utilize the same incision, within the ear area or extended slightly behind the ear into the hairline. After treating deeper neck tissue, the underlying muscle can be tightened and re-positioned backwards. This maneuver restores a desirable youthful appearance. Excess skin is trimmed and patients are delighted that there is less bruising and swelling than they imagined. This benefit is traceable to lifting *deeper* beneath the muscle. There is also less scarring with the procedure I've developed. That's because with more traditional approaches, tension is placed on the superficial layers and the final incision must also bear the weight. As a result, the sutured incision can scar as it heals. By treating deeper tissue, there is less tension placed on the superficial area and the result is a natural and softer look to the jawline and neck, without uncomfortable tightness.

The Hands

You may wonder why I am addressing hands in this section. There's a simple reason and it reflects an important aspect to my personal aesthetic philosophy, especially as it relates facial rejuvenation and the overall natural appearance of any patient. Hands are often overlooked; yet older appearing hands are a certain give away when seen near a beautifully rejuvenated face. This seems unfortunate and unnecessary since some of the same principles used in facelifts can be adapted to achieve youthful hands. Some of the procedures I have adapted with excellent results include a fat transfer from the patient's body to ameliorate thin, volume-depleted hands Also, IPL, or microfractional CO_2 laser can reduce the appearance of wrinkles. Microdermabrasion and chemical peels are effective for more superficial skin blemishes. Some patients may also consider vein sclerotherapy to reduce the appearance of large superficial veins.

Quick Review

While each patient's needs and goals are different, I hope this chapter helps you appreciate how "less" invasive surgery can still deliver superior results. And these results need not be transitory. I've seen many patients enjoy the rejuvenation benefits for many years. Apart from longevity, other benefits include:

♦ Less bruising and swelling since the surgeon lifts deeper beneath the muscle.

♦ A trichophytic incision in the hairline can minimize hair loss and more effectively disguise any scar.

♦ Scars heal better because there is no significant tension on superficial layers and skin.

♦ A natural, softer look without harsh angles and a pulled look.

♦ Youthful definition along the jawline and neck, *without tightness*.

♦ Reduced deflation and restored volume from moving fat and tissue upwards.

♦ The former hollowed, sunken under eye look is gone or diminished, yielding a brighter look.

♦ Reduction of nasolabial folds.

♦ Most patients are able to resume their normal routines within 7-10 days after surgery. 🐦

" A prudent
question
is one-half
of wisdom "

— Francis Bacon

English philosopher, statesman,
scientist, lawyer, jurist and author

Questions

&

Answers

Q. ■ Why Are Facelift Costs So Wide Ranging?

A. ■ Facelift is elective surgery and, as such, fees can vary widely and may or may not include other supplemental surgeries for optimal results. One of the most important factors to determine the cost of the surgery has to do with the individual patient. The amount of facial aging, the medical status of the patient, the degree of sun exposure and habits such as smoking or being overweight will all influence how much work needs to be done. Of course, the patient's cosmetic goals are important as well. Will they need additional work? Would a facelift be pointless in a particular case if a necklift is not done at the same time? These are questions which must be addressed when determining the cost. In addition, a surgeon's cost for facelift surgery is likely based on his or her experience and may include surgeon's fee, surgical facility cost, anesthesia fees, pre-screening medical tests, prescriptions and other incidental costs. The location of the practice, may also be a cost factor.

Q. ■ Will a facelift get rid of all my wrinkles?

A. ■ Facelift is most often performed to "lift" sagging skin, remove skin excess and thus minimize some wrinkles. Some of the deepest lines, such as the frown lines in the forehead (typically improved with a Brow Lift) or the deep lines that run from the nose to the mouth, known as nasolabial folds, may not completely resolve. Further improvement can be achieved with laser skin resurfacing or the use of fillers. Patients with milder aging signs may benefit from Botox or Dysport to control those exaggerated expressions that produce lines such as crows' feet, which are the lines seen at the corners of the eyes. Microdermabrasion or several other conservative procedures are effective in addressing other forms of aging. Some of the best skin smoothers for fine lines, wrinkles, skin discolorations and sunspots can best be addressed by using lasers such as the microfractional CO_2 laser which is one of the most efficient.

Q. ▪ Why should I get a facelift if I can enhance my skin with non invasive methods? What about using procedures such as a "liquid facelift" or a "threadlift"?

A. ▪ A facelift is a type of repair that is meant to lift sagging skin and muscles and restore the architecture of the face. One of my favorite analogies is how one would repair a tent. If you had an old tent that bows in the middle and sags in at the sides, how would you repair it? Sure, you can sew up holes, stretch it more tightly over the frame, pull in slightly or put in a few extra poles to hold it up. At some point, you will need to get a new framework or the tent will not be useful. This is the equivalent to getting the facelift. The repairs and adjustments to the canvas are as far as you can get with the "non-invasive" procedures. The facelift will be the definitive repair so that the skin rejuvenation will look its best.

The "liquid facelift" is a procedure that uses injectibles all over the face to try to mimic the effects of the facelift. But as we have just discussed, you can make changes to the skin, or plump up various parts of the skin, but without fixing the underlying problem, the changes will be short-lived and limited.

The "threadlift" has almost totally been abandoned by many surgeons. The concept was to insert several plastic threads with barbs into the cheek area which would lift the skin and then anchor it higher. It was the equivalent to the extra tent pole to try to hold up the tent. The problem was that eventually the hooks would slip and the threads would slide downwards, become unsightly and uncomfortable and would have to be removed.

Q. ■ **The Mini Lift still gets media coverage. Is it a viable option? Is there a reliable "lunch time" lift?**

A. ■ Few patients are candidates for minor anti aging surgeries. It is virtually impossible to obtain a full beautiful, natural facelift result with a one-hour minimal procedure. It's as simple as that: mini lift, mini results. Many of these types of "minimum" facelifts are superficial skin-only lifts or suture lifts and they don't address underlying sagging tissue and muscle. These procedures do little to address the neck and jowls. They also have a much greater tendency to deteriorate after a short period of time therefore the results are transitory. If it sounds too good to be true, it probably is.

Q. ■ **Will a facelift fix my neck? What about my droopy double chin and jowls? What about the "lunch time" lift?**

A. ■ A facelift may offer some minor rejuvenation to the neck area but strictly speaking, a facelift cannot improve the neck significantly. The surgeries are two distinct procedures. Some patients undergo neck liposuction at the same time as facelift to reduce the fat around the neck or what may be a slight double chin. But liposuction alone has its limits, and it won't fix skin that droops afterwards, if it is a significant amount. This is a separate procedure but often it may be offered in a combination with a facelift, at a discounted rate, if the two surgeries are performed at the same time. A full neck lift improves aging jowls and loose skin in the neck and restores a more clearly defined jaw line.

Q. ■ How much pain will I have?

A. ■ Most patients do not have significant pain. Most patients report some discomfort from swelling or a pulling sensation under the chin. Prescriptions for pain medication are a part of routine postoperative care. Some patients use the prescription medication two to three days after surgery, others feel no need or use Extra Strength Tylenol®. Numbness, especially near the incision lines, is most noticeable in the immediate postoperative period. The area of numbness gets smaller after several months and is rarely permanent.

Q. ■ Will I be in a hospital? Do I go home after cosmetic surgery?

A. ■ We have a Joint Commission accredited facility in both of our offices. We perform our surgeries in our spacious, state of the art operating suites. Most facelifts are done on an outpatient basis and you will need to make arrangements for a responsible adult to drive you home. It is desirable to have a responsible person take care of you for the first 24 hours to help you with ice protocols if they are necessary. Generally, a head wrap dressing is removed after 24 to 48 hours. Sutures require some simple care with antibiotic ointment. In five to seven days, sutures will be removed.

Q. ■ What should I consider before making a decision about cosmetic surgery?

A. ■ The short answer? Gather as much information as you can to make a well-informed decision. Be aware of your motives. What do you hope to get out of your cosmetic surgery? A new lease on life? The answer to all of your problems? No. Are you a perfectionist, one who may fixate on unusually high expectations? Do you believe that you will finally get the promotion or an invitation to a special social event after cosmetic surgery? Unlikely. You could be setting yourself up for disappointment. Cosmetic surgery can enhance your appearance and boost your self-confidence. But it won't necessarily change your looks to match your ideal or cause others to treat you differently. Take some time and think carefully about your expectations. Can you detail your expectations clearly to your surgeon?

All surgery carries some degree of uncertainty. Risks may include the possibility of infection, bleeding, blood clots and adverse reactions to the anesthesia. However, when performed by a qualified cosmetic surgeon, complications will naturally be less frequent and usually minor. Nevertheless, you can reduce your risks by closely following all protocol rules that your surgeon suggests before and after surgery.

Q. ■ Is there an over the counter cure for puffy eyes?

A. ■ Patients must ask me this question every day, albeit wistfully. No, there is no cream that can penetrate the skin, lift your muscles, remove fat from behind the lower eyelids and tack down the lateral end, if necessary. It really is too much to ask from a cream. However, good moisturization of the area is very important to prevent dark circles and fine, wrinkly skin. Some preparations contain witch hazel, also known as, Hamamelis Virginiana or Vernalis, and it is an astringent which temporarily tightens up blood vessels and keeps the eyes looking less puffy for a few hours. For most people who suffer from puffy eyes, this is not a good enough remedy.

Q. Will cosmetic eyelid surgery get rid of crow's feet?

A. Cosmetic eyelid surgery is meant to remove bags under the eyes and the sagging skin of the upper eyelids. It can brighten the appearance by giving the eyes a fresh look. Most fine lines around the eyes will not be affected by cosmetic eyelid surgery. The best method to get rid of crow's feet is to use laser therapy or Botox or Dysport which will smooth out the skin very well.

Q. Will I still need Botox or Dysport if I get my eyes done?

A. You may need Botox or Dysport above your brow, the crow's feet lines and the forehead to get rid of the number 11's if you have them.

Q. ■ Online research has shown me many horror stories about surgery and now I am afraid to get surgery. What can I do about this?

A. ■ It is always difficult to make a decision that involves change. Some people are inherently better with the concept than others. Taking a risk on something you don't understand and can't predict, makes the decision tough. If you interview prospective surgeons and raise your fears and concerns with them, your anxiety will be allayed and hopefully you will be able to make a decision.

Try to be as specific as possible about what frightens you. Is it the anesthesia? In my practice we usually use local anesthesia with IV sedation as needed and this is quite a relief to many of my patients. Is it the risk of surgery? I find that the best way to handle that is to ask to speak with a patient who had the same surgery you are considering and see if the other person can calm your fears. Ultimately, you will have to take a leap of faith and decide if you can live with your decision. Usually, if you think about how relieved and how happy you will be afterwards, you can summon the strength to get the surgery.

Q. ■ Who is the best doctor to do my facial surgery?

A. ■ The best doctor to do your surgery is the one who meets your criteria for credentials and qualifications and who has a vast body of experience combined with artistic talent. You should study before and after pictures and ask questions while looking at them. You should feel as if you have gotten to know your doctor well and you understand his or her philosophy and that he or she has understood your cosmetic goals very well.

Q. ■ I have heard that fat injections around the eyes and in the face will replace the need for surgery. Is this true?

A. ■ Fat will not restore structural support. In the eyelid area, fat can be used in addition to surgery, but only after the underlying area has been reinforced. Aging causes significant weakening of thin structures such as the tissues around the eye. Merely placing fat there may cause further sagging because it is heavy and the tissue underneath is weak. Over six months, fat can be absorbed variably back into the body. Approximately 30% to 70% can be taken back in. Finally, fat can sometimes develop into hardened lumps. These lumps are rather unsightly and surgically very difficult to remove. If you are told that all you need for your eyes and face is a fat injection, make sure you seek other opinions.

Q. ■ Are cheek implants safe?

A. ■ Cheek implants have been performed for decades now. The usual problems with implants are infection or "extrusion" where they come out. When properly placed, infection and other complications are rare. Cheek implants are great for adding a more chiseled look to your face. They are not necessarily used for age related changes. Conversely, submalar implants, which are placed below the cheekbone are used for the face that has suffered volume depletion in this area. This procedure helps to restore the "blooming youth" look that people have in their twenties and thirties.

Q. ■ Is it normal not to be able to close your eyes after surgery?

A. ■ Even if you have swelling, you should be able to close your eyes after surgery. Please consult your doctor if you can't. Certain muscle surgeries such as drooping eyelid surgery (ptosis repair) where the eyelid can be temporarily tightened may result in difficulty closing the eyelids while sleeping. For routine eyelid surgery, it is a myth that you can't close your eyes postoperatively and you need to use a lot of drops for lubrication. Eyes that look good function well. During eyelid surgery, you may have some skin removed, but you should not have had so much skin resected that you can't close your eyes easily.

Q. ■ **How do I know whether I need a blepharoplasty or a browlift? How do I avoid the surprised look?**

A. ■ In general, your doctor should be able to determine which procedure or combination of procedures would better meet your cosmetic needs. Make sure you tell your doctor that you don't want to look perpetually startled. You may have a temporary side effect of a "surprised" expression after certain surgeries, but it should resolve after a few months. Avoiding this side effect is an advantage of the trichophytic browlift.

Q. ■ **I have seen some really bad eye surgeries on celebrities. How do I avoid that look?**

A. ■ Celebrities are not immune to making poor choices. They often live very extreme lives and these habits can have deleterious effects on the healing process. Also, they sometimes depend on the advice of agents or persons who may have a conflict of interest rather than doing their own research and they don't get to study the before and after pictures.

The lesson here is that you should feel confident about the doctor you select , have a connection with him, and trust him to deliver the results you want.

Q. ■ Does insurance cover eyelid surgery?

A. ■ Eyelid surgery is almost never covered by insurance because it is a cosmetic procedure. There are some people who experience vision loss particularly if the eyelids droop to the level of the center of the pupil. Some people have claimed that the surgery improved their vision and have gotten before and after visual field tests to prove it. Despite this medical evidence, insurance companies often deny these claims.

Q. ■ When can I take a shower after surgery?

A. ■ Usually you can take a shower within 48 hours after surgery. Please check with your doctor's office to see if they have specific instructions for you.

Q. ■ **When can I drive after surgery?**

A. ■ We usually advise that people wait for a week so that the stitches have been removed. Before that time, you may be placing ointment in your eyes and your vision will be blurry.

Q. ■ **When can I wear contacts after surgery?**

A. ■ Usually we advise that you wait about 1 to 2 weeks until you have stopped using ointment so that the ointment won't damage the contact lenses.

Q. ■ **When can I wear make up?**

A. ■ You may wear makeup in any area where you have no stitches right away but you should wait 7 days after the stitches have been removed. I recommend mineral based makeup with an SPF for maximal skin protection.

Q. ■ How do I speed up my recovery?

A. ■ The best way to speed up your recovery is to follow the instructions that you received at the doctor's office, get plenty of rest, avoid smoking and eat properly. Do not engage in strenuous activity until you are cleared by your doctor's office.

Q. ■ What about vitamins and supplements?

A. ■ I recommend Vitamin C to all of my patients because it helps the healing process. I have neutral feelings about Arnica ointment and pills. Some of my patients love it but I have not observed a tremendous difference. I tell my patients that they are free to take it if they think it will help them. As for Vitamin E, Ginkoba, Echinacea, and St John's Wort, I recommend that my patients discontinue those supplements for at least 2 weeks. They are all blood thinners and definitely prolong the time in surgery and the healing times afterwards.

231

Q. After how much time can I have sexual relations after a facelift or eyelift?

A. You must check with your doctor because certain positions and levels of activity can affect the healing process. In general, you should probably wait a week because the effects of gravity can make the swelling worse and you may cause too much tension on the incisions. Certain procedures such as a necklift may require that you wait a few days longer than if you had an eyelift.

Q. When can I go swimming after the surgery?

A. You should probably wait about a week until the doctor has cleared you. It is important that your incision is well healed.

Q. ▪ What is the role of facial massage or lymphatic drainage?

A. ▪ Facial massage and drainage may help with reducing swelling, but you should wait at least a week so that the massage will not increase tension and your incisions have healed well.

Q. ▪ What do I tell my family members if I am not ready to talk about the surgery I had? Can I hide this from my significant other?

A. ▪ This is a fairly common question in my practice. I don't recommend that you hide a procedure from your spouse. We do have people who wait until their spouse is away and then get the procedure. Some people change their hairstyle and the spouse will notice that first. Most of the time, the spouse was fearful of the procedure and is relieved after the procedure. Natural aesthetic surgery should leave you still looking like you, so your other family members may not notice and conclude that you look better because you got rest or changed your hairstyle. I do have a patient who told her teenage children who still lived in the house that she was getting over an eye problem and they never asked any other questions again!

Q. ■ **How soon can I drink alcohol after a procedure?**

A. ■ Alcohol is a vasodilator, which means that blood vessels in your face and extremities will dilate and there may be more swelling or bleeding. I recommend that patients wait at least 48 hours, and then drink in moderation so that they don't affect their healing.

Q. What about Recreational drugs or tobacco?

A. Recreational drugs such as marijuana will generate free radicals in your body, that not only speed up the aging process but also slow healing in the same way that smoking does. I would recommend that you don't indulge in these drugs at all during the healing process and seriously reconsider their place in your life if you want to make a commitment to maintaining your youthful appearance.

Q. Should I have someone stay with me during recovery?

A. It is recommended that you have someone stay with you during the healing process at least during the first 24 to 48 hours to help you with your ice protocol and to help you get comfortable.

Q. ■ **When can I exercise or play sports?**

A. ■ Most patients can usually resume this activity about a week later. They should definitely let the doctor know that they are resuming their exercise and describe their regimen so that the doctor can make alternative recommendations, if necessary.

Q. ■ **Can I go back to work sooner than a week if I have a desk job?**

A. ■ You may be able to go back to work sooner if you have a non strenuous job. If you don't have to deal face to face with customers, you may feel more comfortable about returning to work. You will have some bruising and swelling. Some people wear dark glasses and just go, others have been open with their friends and don't mind talking about the swelling afterwards. If you have a more vigorous job, wait at least a week.

Q. ■ **Is the surgery painful? How do I deal with pain?**

A. ■ The surgery should not be painful. If you experience pain during surgery, you should tell the surgeon and pain control will be given until you are comfortable again. After surgery, you may experience some pain for the first day and you will be given pain medication. Usually by the second day, people can use just acetaminophen (Tylenol) and by day five, they usually don't need pain meds anymore. 🖛

OFFICE LOCATIONS

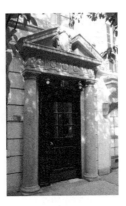

Dr Prasad has two offices in the New York City area. His Manhattan practice is located on the Upper East Side in a discreet, street level brownstone that offers the anonymity that some of our patients seek.

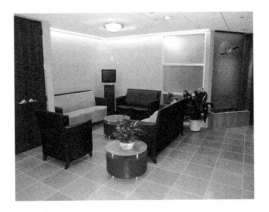

Le Visage Center for Aesthetic Excellence is located in Garden City, New York and is a unique, one stop beauty and image makeover center. There are three entities within the center: Le Visage Cosmetic Surgery, Le Visage Spa and Le Visage Cosmetic Dentistry. Our patients can feel confident that all of their aesthetic goals can be met under one roof and their procedures will be coordinated as efficiently as possible.

ON THE WEB

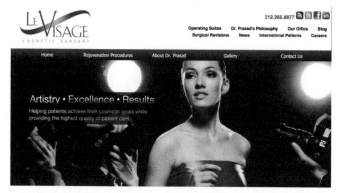

Dr. Prasad's Official Website: www.draprasad.com

www.realfacelift.com

www.eyelifts.com

www.md4hair.com

www.puffyeyes.com

www.coollipodoctor.com

www.levisagecosmetic.com

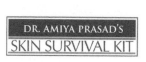

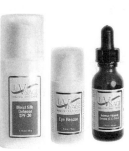

Protect. Restore. Fortify.

SKIN CARE

Le Visage Spa is pleased to present our top of the line, medical grade skin care products that have enhanced and prolonged the cosmetic procedures that we perform. These products were especially formulated by Dr. Prasad and Dr. Pankaj Singh, Le Visage Cosmetic Chief Dentist. Dr. Amiya Prasad's private skin care line, the Skin Survival Kit, is clinically-formulated to improve your skin's tone, texture, and health. Please contact our knowledgeable spa staff for any questions you may have about our product.

The Author — Amiya Prasad, M.D., F.A.C.S.

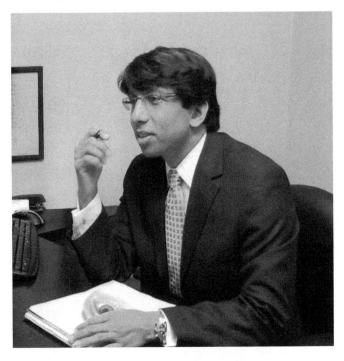

Dr. Prasad has been featured on CBS news, Good Morning America, Fox News, Inside Edition, Channel 11 News, Channel 4 Live at Five and Eyewitness News. He has also appeared in numerous print media such as The New York Times, Haute Living, New York Scene, Avenue, Self, Long Island Business News, Web MD and Health News Digest. Dr. Prasad was one of a handful of cosmetic surgeons featured in the documentary: *Venus Unleashed — The Uncensored History of Plastic and Cosmetic Surgery.*

Learn more about Dr. Prasad and his work at www.draprasad.com, www.realfacelift.com, www.puffyeyes.com and www.eyelifts.com